Overcoming
Chronic Digestive
Conditions

"In recent years, our awareness of the importance of the gut—its structures and the mysteries it contains—has been raised by the arrival of numerous texts on the subject. Most are really useful for reference purposes and for a greater sense of the map and features of the territory within us. Knowledge is useful, but to accelerate our understanding of these mysteries, it is important to have a resource that takes us into the reality rather than simply the theory. Nikki's personal story takes us into that lived reality. It helps to bring the anatomy of the gut to life and, more importantly, to gain some understanding of its relationship to our deepest levels of health and well-being. There are also valuable insights into the potentially long-lasting effects of PTSD and its link to the function of our gut. This book provokes questions and encourages us to look further into this dynamic and fast-evolving area of research and study."

MARGARET ANNE GILL, MBA, CST-D, MCSS,
COAUTHOR OF *THE INNER POWER OF STILLNESS*

"Overcoming Chronic Digestive Conditions is a brilliant read. It's engaging, insightful, educational, and accessible. I would highly recommend it to anyone grappling with their own gut challenges or working in a therapeutic capacity treating those with gut-related health issues. Nikki brings to life through her own experiences how gut health problems are linked to our emotional and physical health, both now and earlier in our lives. The book helps us understand the vicious cycle of cause and effect: how challenges in our emotional and physical health have a knock-on effect on our gut health and how, in turn, the resultant gut challenges further negatively impact us emotionally and physically. I found the practical guidance and strategies immensely powerful as well as the new scientific research. And for those providing hands-on therapy, it will expand their capacity to treat patients, not just with gut disorders but also those with PTSD and neurodegenerative illness, such as Alzheimer's and Dementia. This book never promises to deliver the silver bullet but instead offers a new lens through which to view this complex and fascinating subject."

LINDA MARSH, INTERNATIONAL COACHING
FEDERATION ACCREDITED AND DIRECTOR
AT GRAVITAS MM, LTD.

"This book arose out of Nikki's personal journey toward recovery from PTSD following a diving accident. Along the way, her journey took her into an exploration of her own 'gut feeling.' Her personal journey has become a professional focus. Nikki is using her gathered knowledge to help her own patients as well as educate colleagues and students of many hands-on treatment modalities about this rapidly changing and exciting new area of medical science—the gut/brain connection."

FIONA GILBRAITH, CST-D,
QUALIFIED MEMBER OF THE CRANIOSACRAL SOCIETY

Overcoming Chronic Digestive Conditions

Release the Visceral Layers of Post-Traumatic Gut Disorder

A Sacred Planet Book

Upledger
Institute
International

Nikki Kenward, CST-D, MCSS

Healing Arts Press
Rochester, Vermont

Healing Arts Press
One Park Street
Rochester, Vermont 05767
www.HealingArtsPress.com

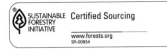

Text stock is SFI certified

Healing Arts Press is a division of Inner Traditions International

Sacred Planet Books are curated by Richard Grossinger, Inner Traditions editorial board member and cofounder and former publisher of North Atlantic Books. The Sacred Planet collection, published under the umbrella of the Inner Traditions family of imprints, includes works on the themes of consciousness, cosmology, alternative medicine, dreams, climate, permaculture, alchemy, shamanic studies, oracles, astrology, crystals, hyperobjects, locutions, and subtle bodies.

Note to the reader: This book is intended as an informational guide. The remedies, approaches, and techniques described herein are meant to supplement, and not to be a substitute for, professional medical care or treatment. They should not be used to treat a serious ailment without prior consultation with a qualified health care professional.

Cataloging-in-Publication Data for this title is available from the Library of Congress

ISBN 978-1-64411-788-0 (print)
ISBN 978-1-64411-789-7 (ebook)

Printed and bound in the United States by Lake Book Manufacturing, LLC
The text stock is SFI certified. The Sustainable Forestry Initiative® program promotes sustainable forest management.

10 9 8 7 6 5 4 3 2 1

Text design and layout by Kenleigh Manseau
This book was typeset in Garamond Premier Pro with Elza and Blacker Pro used as display typefaces
Artwork by Nikki and Andy Kenward

To send correspondence to the author of this book, mail a first-class letter to the author c/o Inner Traditions • Bear & Company, One Park Street, Rochester, VT 05767, and we will forward the communication, or contact the author directly at **nikkikenward.com**.

*

*Dedicated with my love and gratitude always
to my children, Viv and Jon, of whom I am beyond
proud, and who have been the biggest part of
my healing.*

*

Legacy

In dark, quiet moments
I stare down a tunnel
and feel sad

I see myself walking asleep through our lives
Awake only in my love for you
My two blessed children

The gift of family
Embracing, healing
but sometimes undeserved

Cracking open the shell of my pain
I understood the times I failed you

Staring down that tunnel
I am sorry

Seeing you both walk out
And into life
I am proud
and wonder how you became so

And hope the burden of my legacy
Does not touch you too often

You—my highest creation.

Contents

✳

Foreword

Eric Moya, RMT, CST-D, MS/Mfct

Being a very slow eater, I used to get embarrassed to realize that I was still in the middle of my meal when others were done. These days, however, I actually prefer being a slow eater. The more slowly I eat a meal, the more the meal must be affecting me. I savor it.

Eating is the intimate process of taking stuff from the outside and bringing it inside us. Food can hurt us or, if we are careful, food actually becomes our medicine.

A good piece of nonfiction is like a meal that is both nourishing and memorable. We talk about it and share the experience with our friends. We engage in the act of bringing that information into ourselves and digesting it. It takes a while to ingest and digest everything that a work of art has to offer, but doing so transforms us.

This book is like that.

Nikki and I have known each other for about ten years. We have been colleagues as CranioSacral Therapy (CST) instructors. I have been a student of hers, and she has been a student of mine. We've seen each other speak at large conferences, and we have shared meals and collegial social time together. I've always loved her presentation style. When Nikki teaches, she manages to superbly balance being professional and informative with being playful and clear to a lay audience. That is a rare skill and reflects a great deal of insight and personal process. In my own role as the editor and publisher of a magazine about body, mind, and spirit integration, I sought out Nikki as a contributor on the topic of the enteric nervous system, also known as the "gut brain."

Naturally, I originally thought this book would be a companion to the manual therapy course she created for the CranioSacral Therapy community on CST and the enteric nervous system. This book, however, is much larger in scope. It also reveals her personal journey to embody her life process. Better yet, it models the possibilities of undertaking such a personal journey.

This book really is a living analog about the boundary between us and the rest of the world—between our insides and our outsides. It's so easy to forget that our entire digestive system is essentially a long tube that runs through us, which means that our digestive system, one of the most interior of our systems, is technically outside our body. Nikki's book is a body-mind-spirit metaphor for how we navigate and discover ourselves through the contact between our insides and the world around us.

✳

Science has fads and trends. There are many evolving frontiers in therapy that are currently capturing attention and transforming the world of clinical work.

With each new insight or discovery, information spreads outward from the specialists to the rest of us. But some topics catch fire because they resonate with us so much. Perhaps some insight or discovery explains some aspect of our human experience in a new and enticing way or reworks something we always thought to be true. For example, the discovery of neuroplasticity was huge. The idea that our brains can rewire themselves both structurally and functionally from top to bottom based on our experiences was a radical shift. Similarly, with clinical experience and new insights and discoveries about neurobiology, how to work with people who have experienced trauma has radically transformed over the past thirty years. Other insights or discoveries include polyvagal theory, contemporary pain science, the role of glial cells in brain function, and the prevalence and impact of tongue tie and lip tie in infants.

Gut science and the revelation of the enteric nervous system is likely to be another of those new and important frontiers. The discovery that we have a complex nervous system in our bellies—which is able to act independently from the brain and actually influence the brain—is a radically different picture of the nervous system from the one I received in my core therapeutic training around the year 2000. At that time, we believed that our brains were static and unchangeable and that what we had at birth would be all we had to work with for the rest of our lives. We also believed that everything of any importance happened in our heads.

We are still in the infancy stage of understanding what to do clinically with these discoveries about the enteric nervous system. Digestion hasn't carried the attention or the flashiness of working with trauma or brain science, but that's exactly why it needs attention. Our brains tend to grab all of the attention because that is where we think! Yet we have this immense, beautiful, and somewhat quieter body toiling in the background, supporting the brain in its function. In other words, we tend to take the digestive system for granted until it begins giving us trouble.

✳

Nikki's book helps us enter the rich and complex world of the nervous system we have in our abdomen. It helps us understand the beautiful and complicated relationships between our emotions, psychology, and digestion. The book also introduces us to an emerging area of future research, knowledge, and therapeutic skill for body-mind-spirit practitioners. Most of all, it helps us to witness and appreciate the kind of personal transformation that can occur when we listen to our bodies and engage in our own therapeutic processes. Actions speak louder than words, and this book—while also filled with anatomical understanding—is a testimony to letting our personal process take the lead in our education and personal growth.

Don't just read this book. Take the time to digest it and reflect on your own personal history of your gut and your body-mind-spirit process.

Eric Moya, RMT, CST-D, MS/Mfct, is an instructor for the Upledger Institute International. He is publisher and editor of the Idea Crucible, an online magazine based around bodymindspirit integration and therapy.

Acknowledgments

I would like to begin by acknowledging the extraordinary gift given to me and many thousands of others by Dr. John E. Upledger—a gift that has transformed my life and given me decades of fascinating and rewarding clinical practice.

I also want to acknowledge every person who has lain on my treatment table to receive this work. You have taught me so much about body-based process work and shared humanity. I look forward to many more lessons.

To my coach, Lin, for being a hugely encouraging, grounded sounding board who has enabled me to reach clarity when confusion was reigning. I appreciate every minute spent with you.

And to many wonderful and knowledgeable colleagues, family members, and friends—too many to name—who have given me time to brainstorm ideas and who have taken such an interest in this project, an enormous thank you.

And finally, I want to acknowledge the Upledger Institute International, especially Dawn Langnes Shear and Vicki McCabe, for their faith in my work, their support in my development, and their incredible skill in turning ideas into reality.

And finally, *finally,* to my patient husband, Andy, for living through the ups and downs of the whole process with me and still being here! I love you!

Preface

This book is my personal story woven with information and new insights about the amazing nervous system in the gut known as the enteric nervous system. The enteric nervous system is embedded in our esophagus, stomach, and small and large intestines and is often referred to as our "second brain."

It turns out that our second brain plays a much bigger role in our mental, physical, and emotional life than we ever knew. Research over the last few years shows that the second brain can make decisions for itself as well as have complex communication with the brain in the head. In these pages, you will discover the anatomy, function, and complicated wonderfulness of our gut and our second brain.

My intention was never to write a textbook that sits on a dusty shelf for occasional reference. (Apologies to people with enough staying power to properly read textbooks.) I want simply to engage your heart as well as your mind, and I hope that you will want to keep picking up this book and reading it until it is finished. I hope very much that by sharing the experiences of my journey through trauma and its related gut problems, your journey will not be as lonely as mine has often been. I aim to empower you with information and expand your awareness of problems with digestion—including where they might come from and what might be contributing to the whole picture. It would make me very happy if the information, awareness, and hands-on strategies suggested in this book help you experience a more comfortable transition between the two worlds: the world outside as it comes into the world inside the body through the long tube that is your digestive system. This long tube begins in the mouth, then becomes the esophagus, stomach, and small and large intestines. How we experience the transition from the outside in is a fascinating expression of our health.

I do not know of many people with Post-Traumatic Stress Disorder (PTSD) or anxiety who do not have some discomfort and chronic issues in their long tube. I hope the following chapters will answer questions you have had for a long time. You may even end up wondering and reflecting about many new possibilities. I know I have.

In this book, we will go on a journey together to embrace uncertainty and see its value. Let any questions you have float freely in your mind and see what happens. Above all, step into this journey with as much compassion for yourself as you can muster.

If you find the bits about cells and neurology a bit heavy or confusing, you can skip past them to the next bit that intrigues you. I do not wish to overload you, and the chapters contain no multiple-choice tests to see whether you have remembered all the anatomical names, or what they do, or to whom they talk. So relax, take what you need, absorb the gist of the information, and immerse yourself in what interests you now.

NAMASTE,
NIKKI

About Upledger CranioSacral Therapy

Developed by the very extraordinary, late Dr. John E. Upledger, Upledger CranioSacral Therapy has its roots in cranial osteopathy. It is a completely client-centered approach without protocol or agenda. Upledger CranioSacral therapists spend years developing their grounded, blended, neutral therapeutic presence, so they can create a safe, compassionate space for people to experience what they need at that moment. The work is always hands-on and grounded in the tissue of the body. Upledger CranioSacral therapists have, and continue to work on, a thorough knowledge of anatomy and physiology, so they know exactly what is under their hands.

THE CRANIOSACRAL SYSTEM

The head, neck, spine, and everything within make up the craniosacral system, a core system in our bodies. Therapists work with the bones of the cranium (the skull); the vertebrae, including the sacrum and coccyx at the lower end of the spine; the brain and spinal cord (central nervous system and autonomic nervous system); the fluid flowing around and through the craniosacral system; blood and cerebrospinal fluid; the tissue of the brain and spinal cord; and the dural membrane system.

The dural membrane system deserves special mention. Our skull is lined with, and strongly attached to, the dural membrane, which then folds inward to create the curves and arches of our intracranial membrane system. The dural membrane system continues down and out of the skull to line the vertebrae, surround the spinal cord, and eventually blend with the periosteum of the coccyx. It is a little like a balloon with a tail, and the tail is a tube.

The beautiful, strong intracranial membrane system separates and supports the different structures of the brain and contains channels, called venous sinuses, that carry away venous blood and spent cerebrospinal fluid out of the head. This venous blood and spent cerebrospinal fluid then flow through the jugular veins at the base of the skull into the body, where they are to be recycled and recirculated. The degree of tension, patterns of restriction, injuries to, and inflammation of this membrane system have a huge impact on the healthy functioning of our central nervous system and our autonomic nervous system. As well, the cleansing systems in the cranium are adversely affected by a tight membrane system. The intracranial membranes are connected to our brain tissue, so any patterns of tension in the membranes will potentially create patterns of tension in the brain tissue. The venous sinus system can also be compromised by tension in these membranes, and as a result, good fluid flow of venous blood and spent cerebrospinal fluid carrying waste products out of the head can be reduced.

Another important aspect of the dural membrane system is the dural sleeves that branch off each side of the dural tube and carry the spinal nerves away from the spinal cord to their destination, whether that be a muscle or an organ. Tension in one or more of these dural sleeves will compromise the healthy functioning of the nerve it carries.

Emotional and mental stress can cause tension in the dural membrane system. Inflammation (for example, that caused by meningitis or a virus), birth, experiences in the womb, spinal surgery (such as a laminectomy), and surgery elsewhere in the body will impact the fascia, and often that tension will find its way back into the dural system. Many experienced CranioSacral therapists have found that people with autism spectrum disorder have tight dural membranes, which impacts the cleansing of their central nervous system, brain development, and blood flow through and around the brain. Brain injury and concussions also create tension and dysfunction in this system. This tension can lead to such things as headaches and migraines to endocrine disorders, dizziness, foggy head, and memory issues. Good health in this system is of enormous importance for our overall health.

LISTENING TO THE CRANIOSACRAL RHYTHM

The flow of cerebrospinal fluid is a physiological rhythm, like our cardiovascular rhythm or respiratory rhythm. This craniosacral rhythm reflects the fluid's production and absorption in the craniosacral system, which is also part of the healthy environment of the central nervous system. This slow, gentle rhythm is expressed in our connective tissue, our fascia, which runs throughout every part of our body and can be felt by trained hands anywhere in the body. The craniosacral rhythm's quality and vitality can tell us much about what is happening in the body's tissues. Healthy flow of cerebrospinal fluid is an essential component to our health.

Upledger CranioSacral therapists are trained to feel strain and tension patterns in any part of the craniosacral system. Humans are a little like onions in that we build up these patterns in layers over our lifetime—often beginning at birth or even before. Our bodies are very good at adapting to and working around places that don't move so well. But eventually they run out of adaptation resources, and we begin to feel aches or pains or become ill.

CranioSacral Therapy gradually works its way through these layers of tension and adaptation to create healthy fluid flow, freely moving fascia, and a healthy central nervous system. We apply specific gentle techniques, often using the cranial bones as a way into the membrane and fluid systems, to offer the body an opportunity to release tension patterns. We may work all over the body, as the cranial nerves and spinal nerves reach all our muscles, organs, and other tissues. We also work, where appropriate, in the mouth, releasing patterns of restriction and tension in the bones and soft tissues of the palate and jaw. This can be very helpful after dental work and before, during, and after orthodontic work—or when stress has created a pattern of tooth grinding and jaw clenching, for example.

The work involves all aspects of the whole person as needed—physical, emotional, and spiritual. You can probably imagine the kinds of issues we might often see in our clinics: headaches, migraines, all kinds of back and neck pain and problems, neurological problems such as ME or MS, jaw issues, post-surgical problems, and many, many others.

TYPICAL CRANIOSACRAL THERAPY SESSION

In a typical CranioSacral Therapy session, the person lies fully clothed on his or her back on a treatment table or massage couch. The therapist normally begins with his or her hands on that person's feet to feel the craniosacral rhythm and then begins to blend with that person's body tissues to see where it would be most helpful to begin work for that session. He or she might then put his or her hands under different parts of the spine, neck, or head—often with a hand on top of the body too—to follow the biological wisdom of the person and offer the person opportunities to release tension patterns.

SOMATOEMOTIONAL RELEASE

SomatoEmotional Release (SER) techniques are combined with CranioSacral Therapy when appropriate to facilitate release of emotions that may be held in the tissue. SomatoEmotional Release recognizes that our whole history is held in our body. It uses imagery and dialoguing techniques to explore, resolve, and/or integrate any issues. SomatoEmotional release is gentle and respectful.

FOR FURTHER READING

Dr. John Upledger wrote a very accessible introductory volume, *Your Inner Physician and You*,[1] if you would like to know more. There is a recently published introductory book as well, beautifully written by my colleague Kate Mackinnon, *From My Hands and Heart: Achieving Health and Balance with CranioSacral Therapy*.[2]

1
Why Are We Here?

Layers of Tension:
Memories of Being Overwhelmed

It wasn't meant to be like this. Today is Boxing Day (the day after Christmas), and it is the day to start writing my book. This is why we are both here, you and I. I am sitting here with a cold, weak from a horrible sore throat, and my brain is mush. I always planned to start writing today, but I thought I would be fresh and bouncy—not crawling out of a long tunnel of illness.

I cannot ignore my body and take refuge in my intellect. After all, I am telling my story very much through my bodily experience. I want this book to be an honest description of my experiences in the hope that, here and there, some moments will resonate with you, and maybe you will feel less alone.

I will talk later about various theories, but I hope my story will help you to digest these theories at a deeper level. In sharing my story, my goal is to show how each event in my story—moments in which I felt overwhelmed—added another layer of tension or another memory in my gut. Looking back, I see my life divided into chunks—sometimes by events (marriages, broken hearts, house moves, professional milestones), sometimes divided by me deliberately. In order to get through the journey's tougher parts, when the whole journey seemed overwhelming, I would say to myself, "I just need to get through the next two weeks and see if I feel better, and if not, I'll look at my options." Sometimes those options were very final. Fortunately, there has never been a two-week period where things have not improved in my mind, heart, and body. So here I am, feeling pretty terrible, but somehow ready to share a few of these tidbits with you and see where that takes us.

The journey will probably take us into the gut in the end—at least that is where I am intending on heading; but first I invite you to meet some of my memories, the memories that began all this.

So many moments are clamoring for my attention that at first I don't know where to start. But I think it has to be the diving accident, which occurred in 2003. This memory always jumps up and down in my brain and calls to me. Nothing has ever been quite right since then, although in other ways, things have been more right than they were before.

There is nothing like facing your own mortality and coming back from the brink. You see how pointless most of life really is, and yet, you become equally anxious, worried more about the pointless things, even though you can now see how pointless they are.

Memory: Holiday in Ireland

Let me set the scene. I am on holiday on the West Coast of Ireland. It is summer, but the sea is still very cold. I have been scuba diving many times before, but only in the balmy waters of the Red Sea, so I do not know how different this will be both mentally and physiologically. The dive leaders seem to be more interested in selling the dive than explaining these differences to me and considering whether the dive is appropriate for me. They say they will look after me and that I need not worry. As a result, I find myself sitting in a little boat with an outboard engine along with a few other people, traveling out across a deep blue sea in the sunshine, feeling anxious. I am wrapped up in a semi-dry suit, diving shoes, and gloves, with a balaclava on my head. All this gear is new to me. I have only dived in warmer waters where nothing but a short wetsuit was required.

As we approach the dive site, I continue to ignore the quiet voice inside me asking if I am sure I want to do this dive, especially in cold water wearing equipment I have never worn before. I remember answering that voice, "I will be fine; the dive leaders will take care of me; I do not need to worry." The dive masters make fun of my anxiety and ask if I am afraid of being a little cold. Perhaps that makes me more determined to go ahead and ignore the little voice whispering in my ear, "Are you sure you should do this dive?"

Descent

Once we are all tanked up, we roll backward over the edge of the boat into the water, one by one, to begin our descent. I roll off the edge of the boat, watching sea and sky change places—something I have done many times before—swapping the freedom of air and sun, through loud water crashing, for the isolating silence of the sea.

I begin my descent. There is a rope line to guide us since there are no visual reference points—just a sheer dark rock face a little way from us, off to one side, and the deep, cold, turquoise water. The other divers are disappearing beneath me very quickly.

The sea becomes a deep aquamarine and then a deep green with nothing to hang my gaze on—no coral, no rocks, no sand—just endless cold blue water above, in front, behind, and below.

I begin to feel dizzy and unsure of any certain orientation. What is up and what is down becomes confusing.

Locked in my own world with my own breath as a score for my performance, I hear my inhalations becoming ragged in my ears. I struggle to keep up the pace, pausing to clear my ears every few meters, and adjusting my buoyancy to drop down and down and down and down. I remember feeling that descent as an enormous rush, a race to the bottom. I am afraid I am going to be left behind, hanging in the blue with no one near me and nothing around me.

I arrive at the bottom to find the others already there. I am gulping my air, trying to calm down, and scared of what might lie ahead.

The dive master signs to me immediately to tighten my weight belt. A semi-dry suit is thick at the water surface but gets squashed as you descend to deeper waters and deeper pressures. My weight belt has become loose. Were it to fall off, I would rush to the surface and damage my lungs, as well as possibly get the "bends." She is right. I know I must do this, but I am feeling overwhelmed by the descent and unable to figure out this task. In order to tighten my weight belt, I need to make my body horizontal, facing the bottom, so that when I undo the belt to tighten it, it will not fall off. Even though I know this, my body is already stressed and my brain is screaming, "I can't do this!" I tip myself forward, begin to open the buckle, and pull the belt a little tighter. I don't remember whether I succeeded in tightening the belt at all. In the end, that was to become irrelevant.

If this starts to sound muddled, know that I am resisting my natural urge to make the accident sound less than it was. Whether you feel I am making a fuss or if you are upset by my experience, my aim is to share the reality of what happened. Just as I am sitting here remembering all this with a bad cold and a hot lemon and honey drink by my side—this is my reality.

Regulator Filled with Water

I notice that time begins to behave in a peculiar way, and my senses are stretched to the breaking point. The regulator in my mouth quickly fills up with water during the slow-motion tipping of my body from vertical to horizontal. I find it surprisingly difficult to part water on either side of me as my body leans forward. I do not expect this mouthful of water. I feel my heart thump. I remember my drills and blow into my regulator to drive out the water.

Somehow, I now shift into a surreal world, a bit like the one in which Alice in *Alice in Wonderland* found herself. I am transported into a nightmare from which I cannot wake up. My heart is thumping loudly in my ears. My brain is wracked for ideas but unable to think. The water is relentlessly cold, blue, and unending all around me. Sixty feet of sea is pressing down on top of me. My regulator refills with water. Gathering all the breath I have left in my lungs, I breathe sharply out again to clear it, but immediately, it again fills with salty water.

Zero Options

It amazes me that I can run out of ideas so rapidly—that in a single moment my options are reduced to zero. I have been desperate to take a breath for what seems like a very, very long time, but the regulator is full of the sea. All of my remaining breath I have used up in my attempts to clear my regulator, the piece of equipment that was keeping me alive.

Can you imagine what it would be like if, just as you were about to thankfully take a big gulp of air, you couldn't? I am taken beyond that point so many times, and my lungs and whole body feel like bursting open. I know I cannot ascend rapidly to the surface, as I have no air to breathe out, and in any case, I am not sure my brain is capable of working out how I might do that. Writing this, my breathing is becoming difficult; my heart is thumping; and my gut is gurgling.

Pain Everywhere

I am hanging there in the water—adrenaline pumping through my body, fear building in every cell, panic pounding in my chest—until my body takes over.

It breathes. It has no choice. I can no longer control it. But it breathes in seawater.

I feel the cold, dense saltiness of the water forced down the back of my throat into my windpipe. My brain rapidly computes this as a disaster. The water is bubbling inside me; from somewhere pain is rising; and, of course, I still have no air. Panic and fear meet head on in an explosion of terror and the stark realization that I am drowning.

So this is what drowning feels like. How odd. I can remember clearly having that thought.

All I can feel is cold water in and around me, pain everywhere. All I can hear is some strange gurgling from my throat. My body takes over again, rushing in with its last hope, its last idea for survival. It is as if a hand suddenly closes around my throat and with great force. My body is strangling itself in an attempt to stop the seawater from reaching too far into my lungs. Every muscle in my throat and neck goes into a brutal spasm to stop the tide filling my lungs. Now, the only sound I hear is an odd squeaking in my throat. I think it is my larynx. It is a strange sound. *So this is what suffocating is like,* I think.

There is no capacity in any cell of my body to feel more panic or terror, so my whole self—mind and body—moves beyond that. I find myself in a calm, empty place filled only with the sound of my asphyxiation and a deep, heart-breaking sorrow that I am leaving my two children too soon. I am waiting to die. I know it will be soon. Helpless, without hope, suspended between life and death, between two worlds, I am drowning. I am dying. Everywhere is blue; everywhere is cold; I am alone; everyone else is somewhere else; no sound except the squeaks from my throat; no sound of breath; floating like a dying fish in an enormous tank.

Lung and Heart Damage

It is at this point that I become vaguely aware of the dive master. She has noticed me, and realizes I am in trouble. She comes toward me and is staring into my eyes. I don't know what she sees there. She offers me her spare breather, but as I am in spasm, I am unable to breathe from it, so she holds it just in front of my face. I see the bubbles of air coming out in front me rise up through the cold water. I feel completely detached and think *What does all this have to do with me?* Some part of me is hanging onto consciousness.

Grabbing hold of my buoyancy control device, she takes me rapidly up to the surface. I cannot breathe out as we ascend.

I break the surface of the water, and my body stops strangling me. I gasp for air, spitting out water, gasping again and again, yelling, "I can't breathe! I can't breathe!"

I am heaved onto the boat, my tank removed as well as my buoyancy control device and balaclava, and I am given oxygen. My whole body is in shock, shaking.

Because I could not breathe out, my lungs were damaged during the quick ascent. My heart had not had oxygen for a long time, so it was damaged too. What had happened to my mind would only be revealed in the coming year. Sadly, the dive master does not take me to the hospital and instead tells me I will be okay. On the one hand I believe her, as she has so much experience, and on the other hand I don't believe her, but I do not have the capacity to advocate for myself at that moment. I would later find that lack of early treatment damaging.

That night I wake up in the middle of the night with my whole body shaking and feeling sick and wobbly inside. This is to become a familiar set of sensations. I make some tea and go back to bed but do not sleep much.

Waiting for Things to Improve

Two days later I fly home to England, still feeling very strange. I call a friend who teaches diving locally and tell him what happened. He asks me to meet him for a cup of tea, so I drive over immediately. He is very concerned, and he suggests I go straight to the local emergency department. I am alarmed but trust his judgment and head straight for the hospital, where they are bemused, as a scuba accident survivor is not something they see very often.

The doctors do various tests and tell me my lungs will probably mend in a couple of months. They suggest perhaps I should find a diving chamber. I decide I probably don't have the "bends," so I go back to working in my clinic and wait for things to improve. Sure enough, after two months, my lungs do feel much better, so I feel I am now 100 percent okay and can move on. I even plan a trip to the Red Sea over Christmas—now a couple of months away—to do some more diving.

Room Spinning

Christmas arrives, and I arrive in Sharm el Sheikh. I book my advanced PADI diving course. But the night before my first dive, everything changes.

That night I dream about the dive the next day. In my dream everything goes wrong during the dive, and I am filled again with panic and terror. I wake in the night and the room is spinning. I close my eyes and go back to sleep. In the morning, I open them, and everything is still spinning. I feel very sick and lurch for the loo, where my bowels empty themselves rapidly. I do not know what is happening, but I know I cannot dive that day. I go back to bed.

The spinning settles down a little, as long as I move slowly and carefully and do not lie down flat anywhere. Inside, my head feels dizzy and my whole world seems uncertain. I feel I am not connected to this real world but about to float off to some other place or dimension and that I have no control over this. I do very little for the rest of my short stay in "Sharm" and am relieved to fly home.

Anxiety Grows

The dizziness does not wear off, and the accompanying anxiety grows. I begin to notice heart palpitations and odd rhythms. My sleep is disrupted by these thumps and tumbles and somersaults in my chest that are usually followed by cramping in my gut, loose bowel movements, and nausea. After a day or two, my guts settle, and I am left with a big headache. Then the whole cycle begins again. I start to look thin and pale, with large black rings round my eyes. I have no energy and increasingly want to stay at home. I go to see my doctor, who gives me vertigo medication, tells me to stop driving, and sends me to a neurologist.

My world becomes smaller and smaller. Being at home and walking to shops and my clinic are all I do. The neurologist sends me for a CT scan to see if I have had a stroke. At our follow-up appointment, he dismisses me brusquely, saying there is nothing neurologically wrong with me and I need to go see a cardiologist. By this time, I look terrible and have become so dizzy with heart rhythms that I nearly pass out. Nausea and loose bowels are familiar to me but never my friend. I am exhausted and restless at night—feeling isolated and confused but too ill to really know what to do next.

I cannot lie down to sleep, as I feel I will float off into an empty, black place far away and never come down again. It is a terrifying sensory experience. In the morning, I have to dodge the shower with my face and mouth or my whole body goes into a panic and I cannot breathe. As I am making breakfast for my children and preparing to go to my clinic, I often have to lie down for a few minutes. I feel so weak that I hold on to the walls of houses as I walk to work with unsteady legs. When I begin driving again six weeks later, I am so anxious on the roads that driving becomes terrifying. I take my son to tae kwon do on a frosty evening and am so scared on the way home that, when I finally return, I sit sobbing beside my radiator in the living room, wondering how I will get back in the car to pick him up. I stop going out socially. I feel anxious about everything.

Late-Onset Post-Traumatic Stress Disorder

I do not know it yet, but this is chronic late-onset Post-Traumatic Stress Disorder, and it hits me like a massive truck, nearly wiping me out. I feel so ill that I use some savings to go to see a cardiologist privately. I cannot wait any longer for help. The cardiologist does an echocardiogram and puts monitors on me for a few days to see what is happening. Many of my symptoms align with decompression illness, which of course makes sense, as I had not been breathing on my ascent. He sends me to see a colleague of his to see if he thinks I would still benefit from going into a dive chamber.

Very kindly, his colleague makes time for me that day and does not even charge me. He is compassionate and very thorough, but he feels it is too late for me to benefit from the decompression chamber. I am disappointed and angry that I was not taken to a chamber as soon as I had had the accident. My cardiologist tells me that my heart seems structurally undamaged, but there are rogue cells all over the heart that are firing off the three different arrhythmias I am experiencing: tachycardia, premature ventricular contractions, and premature atrial contractions. This means I cannot have a cardiac ablation to correct the arrhythmias, which only works on identifiable and isolated groups of cells. My only option seems to be anti-arrhythmia drugs. I work my way through three different drugs in the next nine months, all designed for people with major heart problems. They all turn me into a zombie whom my friends barely recognize. The arrhythmias remain the same. My cardiologist sends me one more prescription, and when I read about the accompanying challenging side effects of the drug he is recommending, I decide I cannot take any more drugs and put it in a drawer.

Beginning of Recovery

I ask a consultant friend for advice. She knows a cardiologist that she highly recommends. He turns out to be the beginning of my recovery. Kind and knowledgeable, he redoes all the tests, echo-cardiogram, and twenty-four-hour monitoring. His conclusions are the same, except that he agrees that I can tackle this without drugs. He recognizes the high anxiety I am now experiencing and the trauma I have been through. He says one thing that helps me massively: "Don't try to be the person you were before the accident." And I realize that is what I have been aiming for. But of course I am different. The experience has changed everything.

I now feel I am on a journey to discover who I am. I can now grieve for the person I have lost as well. I am very sad, but I also feel a tiny germ of curiosity about the future. Somehow my whole energy has shifted to a more useful place, a more real place that is simultaneously a relief and a daunting challenge. How much of this experience will I be able to integrate and who will that make me? How will my body recover from this trauma and what lasting memories will it retain?

I hesitate to talk to anyone about my experiences because I do not know any other person who has nearly drowned. But I am gradually becoming aware that all the physical and emotional symptoms—nausea, dizziness, anxiety, body in fight or flight most of the time, cramping and overactive bowels, social anxiety, insomnia, flashbacks, intrusive memories, and a profound sense of isolation—add up to chronic late-onset Post-Traumatic Stress Disorder. My doctor agrees and is incredibly compassionate. I take action and start having regular acupuncture, Upledger CranioSacral Therapy, and psychotherapy. All my therapists agree that my problem is PTSD, and that helps me accept my situation. I also take up yoga.

The New Me

My progress is incredibly slow, but gradually, the heart arrhythmias diminish. Over three years, I manage to get rid of them for the most part. My other symptoms become less intense. I am drug free and beginning to live my life again. I love yoga with a passion. The first six months, I could barely bend down in any asana without experiencing great dizziness and distress that would require me to stand up and walk around my mat, rubbing my temples before I could carry on. Now I can do headstands and handstands and love being upside down. That is the part of the new me that I love.

The parts I still struggle with are the anxiety and gut issues. I know they are closely linked and they can be debilitating. I still have that sense of isolation. These are the parts of the new me that I love less. Every day, for a long time, I would read *The Perfect*

Storm—a story with a few pages describing someone else's near drowning—just to feel less alone with my experience. It is as if part of me will always be between two worlds—coming back to this world but still partly attached to another place and time, unable to forget or leave that event completely behind.

Two Weeks at a Time

For years, my mantra became "Two weeks at a time—my life with PTSD." When I became very depressed about the accident's emotional and physical residue, I would tell myself that if I could just get through the next two weeks, then I had permission to end my life. By the end of the two weeks, things would usually change for the better, and I would remain in this world. Would I have committed suicide? I hope and believe not—for the sake of my family. Did I sometimes want everything to end? Yes, I did.

I very rarely share what it feels like, physically and emotionally, inside me because there does not seem to be any hope of anyone understanding or of that sharing helping me. At the time, it felt like sharing would be more likely to push people away. Alternatively, I feel that others will feel like I am exaggerating and that the PTSD is not real. I prefer not to try to explain it at all than experience someone I trust belittle it or imply that I should be over it by now. So I stay silent most of the time. The price I pay for this silence is the energy it takes to hide part of me—a separation from most people in my life and often a feeling of despair. For years, I felt a deep sense of isolation.

The sense of empathy, shared humanity, and compassion for others that I bring to the people in my practice and in my personal life has been an enormous gift, a gift that came from working through this experience.

The part of me that seems to hold the trauma so deeply, yet is so hard to reach, is my digestive system. So many stories are here. How can I hear them? I feel so disconnected from this part of myself. For more than ten years this remained a real weakness. Or that is how I have always viewed it. Perhaps my digestive system just needs me to listen more carefully to what it is trying to tell me. It affects everything—sleep, energy, happiness—and I just become so bored with feeling the same way, with explaining to people that my tummy isn't feeling great, an explanation that makes light of something that really isn't light at all. It is a dark and desperate place that I do not understand. In the last few years, I have begun to hear the messages more clearly. I have come further away from shame and frustration with myself and my body and moved closer toward acceptance, compassion, and self-care.

✳

JOURNEY INTO THAT DARK PLACE

This book is the story of my journey into that dark place. A place that itself is between two worlds. The outside world comes into our inside world through our mouth and down the long tube, until it leaves us out the other end (fig. 1). How do we respond to this? Do we embrace it or shrink away from it? Are we scared and anxious? Do we brace ourselves? Is the whole experience relaxed and comfortable and welcoming? Or does our body in this transitional place tighten and tense itself for the invasion? How does our physical and emotional history impact our response to the outside world's coming in? What can we do to influence that in some small way?

This is why we are here, you and I, on this page. This is the story of my life, as well as the story of all our lives in some ways.

I am here because I realized that by not talking about my

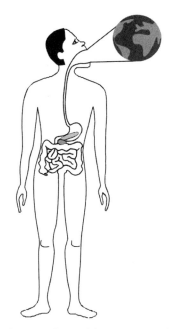

Figure 1. The outside world coming inside.
How do we respond?

Post-Traumatic Gut and associated struggles for fear of being judged or silenced, I was actually part of the problem. Not talking about the bowels and not talking about mental and emotional health issues is what makes these topics taboo. Talking about them in the same breath is an even bigger taboo.

Why are you here? Perhaps something is already resonating with you? I hope some of this will be a tiny torch for you to shine on your own digestive system to begin to understand how it works, or perhaps a tiny ear trumpet to help you listen a little more attentively to its messages today and from the past. The more connected we all are to our felt sense of our inner world and how that responds to the outer world, the more empowered we are to help ourselves become healthier and happier, and the better we understand how to take care of ourselves.

With that in mind, I have included a tummy tracker page in the appendix of this book. It asks: "If your gut could make a face right now, what would it look like?" This is a question to keep in mind as you read this book. I hope what I've written inspires you to listen to your gut more often and begin a journey toward better health and increased happiness.

2
Our Life in Our Body

There are very simple ways of building your felt sense of your inner world, or your interoception, as you begin to search for the stories in your own second brain. When you have a few minutes and can be undisturbed, explore these practices. One way is to put your hands on your abdomen while lying down or seated in a comfortable position—wherever feels right for this moment—and listen with them, without judgment or analysis. Notice how your body feels under your hands, and notice what pops up into your awareness as you do this. If what pops up seems bizarre or does not make sense, so much the better; it is probably from a deeper place than anything more logical or rational. Notice how soft and relaxed or tense and stiff the tissues feel. Pay attention to any sense of fluid flow, energetic flow, or temperature differences. Perhaps there are some places that feel numb. Take a few moments to ponder this; make a note of what you experience, and continue.

If you would like to and feel ready to progress, the next step is to visualize all the layers in the gut that you have your hands on. By doing so, you will get more information about what is happening and where the tension patterns are held most deeply. We will explore these layers shortly. In order to get the most from this idea, you should also be familiar with the basic anatomy of the gastrointestinal tract.

BASIC ANATOMY OF THE GASTROINTESTINAL TRACT

The gastrointestinal tract is a long tube from our mouth—where we invite and receive the outside world inside of us—to our anus. Nine meters long in a body at autopsy (but a little shorter in a living body, as it is held in a degree of tone and tension), it can be thought of as our largest external surface. The large, hollow organs of the gastrointestinal tract or the alimentary canal (fig. 2) contain layers of muscle that enable their walls to move. This movement of the organ walls, called peristalsis, propels food and liquid through the gastrointestinal tract and mixes the contents inside each organ. Peristalsis looks like an ocean wave traveling through the muscle as it contracts and relaxes.

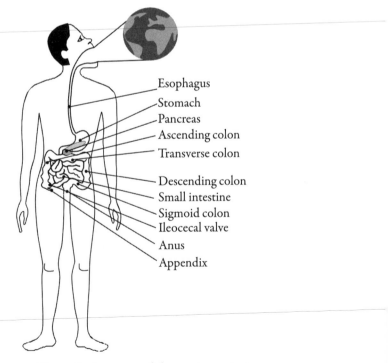

Esophagus
Stomach
Pancreas
Ascending colon
Transverse colon

Descending colon
Small intestine
Sigmoid colon
Ileocecal valve
Anus
Appendix

Figure 2. Anatomy of the gut in context.

Peristalsis has an interesting and almost comical story of discovery. In 1917, pharmacologist Ulrich Trendelenberg did an experiment in which he put a piece of guinea pig intestine in an organ bath and blew into it through a J-shaped tube. Much to his surprise, it blew back! Completely unattached to anything else, it clearly had the reflex circuits required to respond autonomously. This was the amazing discovery of peristalsis, the ocean wave that carries along our food and our experience through our long tube. This incredible experiment showed that the gut had its own nervous system that did not need any input from the central nervous system to act and react. But somehow Trendelenberg's name was lost from scientific study. In 1921, English scientist John Newport Langley published his book *The Autonomic Nervous System: Part 1*. It included this information and named the three aspects of the autonomic nervous system: sympathetic, parasympathetic, and enteric. Yet it has only been in the last ten years or so that the enteric nervous system has been recognized as a third branch of the autonomic nervous system.

JOURNEY THROUGH THE GASTROINTESTINAL TRACT

Let's take a simple journey with our food down the long tube. First of all, we put food and liquid into our mouth, where digestion begins as we chew. This is a very important first stage in successful digestion and absorption. Our teeth and the enzymes in our saliva enable us to begin breaking down food to prepare it for the rest of its journey. Ideally, we would chew at least twenty-five times for each mouthful; if we are ill, fifty times for each mouthful, according to many traditional medicines and modern nutritionists. When I began to chew every mouthful twenty-five times, I found something magical seemed to happen at around twenty to twenty-five chews: everything in my mouth became a liquid, ready to swallow.

When we swallow, we push our food into the esophagus, the muscular tube that carries food and liquid from the mouth to the stomach. Once swallowing begins, the process becomes involuntary, no longer under our control. Digestion is then under the control of the esophagus and the two brains, the one in the head and the one in the gut. (I am tempted here to say three brains and include the microbiota, which are a huge part of this process.)

As food approaches the closed sphincter, the muscle of the upper part of the stomach, it relaxes to allow the food to enter. The lower esophageal sphincter, a ring-like muscle where the esophagus meets the stomach, opens to let food and liquid into the stomach.

The muscle of the lower part of the stomach mixes swallowed food and liquid with gastric juice, a thin and strongly acidic, almost-colorless liquid secreted by glands in the stomach's lining. The pyloric sphincter then allows the resulting mixture, called "chyme," to flow into the small intestine.

More mixing! The muscles in the small intestine mix the chyme with digestive juices from the pancreas, liver, and intestine. Nutrients are also absorbed through its walls into the bloodstream, and blood delivers the nutrients to the rest of the body via the liver.

The remains of this digestive process include undigested parts of food and old cells from the gastrointestinal tract lining. The wave of peristalsis, which the layers of muscle create, push these waste products into the large intestine through the ileocecal valve, which opens to allow it all through and then closes again. The large intestine, or bowel, absorbs water and any remaining nutrients and turns the waste from liquid into stool. The rectum stores this waste until it leaves the body through the anus during a bowel movement.

Remember, because this large hollow tube is full of the outside world, we might think of it as our largest external surface. The gastrointestinal epithelial barrier that lines the intestines and bowel hovers between two worlds, the outside world and the world inside our body. Perhaps it is one place where our two worlds can communicate and find a meeting place, negotiating for our health—physical, mental, and emotional.

ENTERIC NERVOUS SYSTEM

The enteric nervous system is embedded in the walls of the long tube and is a complicated center for processing huge amounts of data from the lumen (the hole running through the middle of the tube), its contents, the epithelial barrier, and the response of our brain in the head.

The enteric nervous system communicates with the brain in the head via the vagus nerve, as well as through our hormones and our stress response systems, such as the reticular activating system–hypothalamus-pituitary axis. It has all the neurotransmitters that we have in our central nervous system—at least thirty of them. The enteric nervous system sends many more messages to the brain in our head than the brain in our head sends to the second brain. This communication system is referred to as the gut-brain axis. It turns out we have a brain in our gut as well as in our head.

The enteric nervous system as such was discovered in the small intestines of dogs in the nineteenth century by physiologists Bayliss and Starling. In the late nineteenth century, the two main plexi of the enteric nervous system were discovered. Leopold Auerbach, a German anatomist and neuropathologist, discovered the myenteric plexus between the two muscular layers of the esophagus, small intestine, and large intestine. Auerbach's plexus, as it is also called, has motor output that largely controls the pushing movements of the gastrointestinal tract, but it also has some sensory nerves. It has both sympathetic and parasympathetic input from the autonomic nervous system. German anatomist George Meissner found the smaller submucosal plexus (also called Meissner's plexus), near the lumen or space in the middle of the tube.

Nerve fibers from the larger Auerbach's plexus perforate the circular muscle layers to create the smaller Meissner's plexus under the mucosa. Meissner's plexus has both motor and sensory functions. It is also connected to both sympathetic and parasympathetic aspects of the autonomic nervous system, as well as innervates, or supplies nerves to, the secretory part of the mucosa and so can make glands secrete a substance like mucus or serous fluid. Meissner's plexus also innervates the epithelial layer—that layer of tissue closest to the lumen—as well as innervates the muscularis mucosa. The larger Auerbach's plexus extends upward into the esophagus, whereas the smaller Meissner's plexus does not. It is found mainly in the small intestine, where its sensory neurons can feel what is happening.

These two nerve plexuses, as well as the other nerve fibers and nerve cells in the gut, make up the enteric nervous system, or second brain. Let's see if we can illuminate the recent discoveries that suggest how the brain in the head may have evolved from the second brain and evaluate how this connection may strongly influence our emotional and mental health.

ENTERIC NERVOUS SYSTEM EVOLUTION AND EMOTIONAL/MENTAL HEALTH

It is thought that there is a close connection between the development of our enteric nervous system and the evolution of early parts of the brain, the limbic regions, which are responsible for our emotions, our intense life experience, the autonomic nervous system, vagus nerve, and the reticular activating system. The enteric nervous system is not a uniquely human or even mammalian system. Similar systems are found throughout the animal kingdom, including in insects, snails, and even marine polyps. It is thought that the nerve ganglia that created the primitive brain of worms and, eventually, higher mammals, came from more primitive but homologous enteric nerve circuits. This shows a close connection between our enteric nervous system and early parts of the brain, the limbic regions.

Thus, neural circuits and communication systems have evolved over time. Optimal responses, such as whether to approach or withdraw from the challenges presented by our internal environment (for example, the luminal environment), may well have been incorporated into the central nervous system during evolution. Our long digestive tube, as we now recognize, is the largest external surface of our body, so these responses could be said to have evolved to react to our external environment as well.

In human babies developing in the womb, the enteric nervous system is born from cells that travel from the neural crest of the embryo, along the vagus nerve, to find their home in the gut. These neural crest cells grow up into neurons and glia during the embryo's development and continue to do so in early postnatal life (up to three months after birth). It takes at least three weeks for them to reach and populate the gastrointestinal tract. It is the longest journey undertaken by baby neurons anywhere in the body. Interestingly for our work in CranioSacral Therapy, these cells that travel the neuraxis (the axis of the central nervous system) to colonize the gut come from the vagal and sacral parts of the neuraxis, thus creating a close developmental connection between the enteric nervous system and the autonomic nervous system.

Based on these close connections with limbic and autonomic regions of the brain, the enteric nervous system can be looked at as a peripheral extension of the limbic system into the gut, where it is exposed closely to our complex internal and external environment in the lumen, which can include powerful mechanical, chemical, emotional, and microbial influences. When I discovered these connections, I could see the huge implications for our emotional and mental health. Alternatively, the limbic and autonomic system can be viewed as an encephalized portion of the enteric nervous system.

Either way you want to think of it, this has all the same implications: these two parts of us have been connected through time. Is knowing this a way we can begin to become aware of the enormous emotional memory component of gut issues and its direct line to the limbic system (fig. 3)? Through this awareness, we can move forward in our growth toward optimal health.

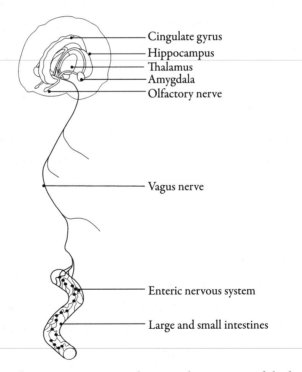

Figure 3. Evolutionary connections between the anatomy of the limbic system in the brain and the enteric nervous system (or second brain) in the gut.

Figure 3 illustrates the connection between the enteric nervous system in the gut and the limbic portions of the brain. Together, this can be seen as the gut-brain axis, originating from our evolutionary journey when the limbic system was created out of the development of the enteric system. As CranioSacral therapists, these old evolutionary journeys can be felt in the body when we are treating a patient.

Our second brain buzzes with activity throughout our gut. Sitting here now, I can feel mine responding to my plans for the day and responding also to the porridge I just had for breakfast this morning!

LAYERS OF SMALL INTESTINE

Do you recall when I told you near the start of this chapter that I would discuss the layers of the gut so that you could gain information from them and come to understand the tension patterns they hold? Now that you understand the basic anatomy of the gut, how it evolved, and its connection to the limbic system and autonomic nervous system, I will take you on a more detailed look at the layers in which Auerbach's and Meissner's plexuses are found: the amazing layers of the small intestine where absorption of nutrients takes place. We will start from the outside and work our way through the layers, moving inward (fig. 4; p. 26).

Mesentery

We will start by looking at the mesentery, the outermost layer and covering of the small intestine and bowel. The mesentery is an extension of the serosa and adventitia. A most extraordinary structure, the mesentery has recently been identified as an organ in its own right (upgraded from being considered four separate pieces of connective tissue).[3] If you were to imagine the mesenteric organ as a

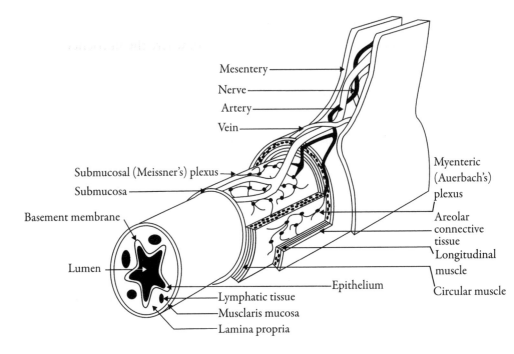

Mesentery

Nerve

Artery

Vein

Submucosal (Meissner's) plexus

Submucosa

Basement membrane

Lumen

Myenteric (Auerbach's) plexus

Areolar connective tissue

Longitudinal muscle

Circular muscle

Epithelium

Lymphatic tissue

Muscularis mucosa

Lamina propria

Figure 4. Cross section, through the small intestine, showing the enteric nervous system (or second brain) in layers of mesentery.

dress fabric, as nineteenth-century physician Worthington Hooker suggests, it would be like a ruffle around the puffed edges of the small intestines. Even Leonardo da Vinci knew about the mesentery and drew it with great accuracy.

The mesentery is formed from the double fold of the peritoneum (a continuous transparent membrane made of connective tissue [fascia] that lines the abdomen and surrounds the organs [viscera]). It is coated in mucus to prevent any friction damage from the intestine's rubbing against other tissue. The mesentery connects the small intestine and bowel to the back wall of the abdomen, holding it all in place. Without this, our carefully curved and folded gut would lie in a tangled heap in our pelvis. The mesentery carries a blood, lymph, and nerve supply to the tissue of the gut, through its two layers, and carries the nutrients from the gut back to the liver through the blood and lymph vessels in the villi, where the nutrients can be stored and turned into useful energy.

The new knowledge that the mesentery is a single organ will eventually help many people with abdominal disease. It will also help the hands of Upledger CranioSacral therapists, and of other bodyworkers, work with people who come to them for help, as the mesentery can also hold tension or strain patterns.

Before proceeding on our journey to the center of our personal universe, how can we as bodyworkers work with the mesentery? If we are working on someone with one hand on top of the abdomen and one hand underneath, we can listen very carefully to the mesenteric organ and feel for any tension and restriction patterns there. If we are Upledger CranioSacral therapists, we can listen to the craniosacral rhythm as well and notice any Significance Detector activity (when the craniosacral rhythm stops; see p. 83). If we are working on ourselves with both hands placed on top of our body, why not send our intention through to the mesenteric organ underneath and listen from there?

Longitudinal Muscle—Outer Layer of the Muscularis Externa

Dropping in one more layer, we find the longitudinal muscle, one of the muscles of peristalsis, that pushes food through our gut in waves.

Auerbach's (Myenteric) Plexus

Then we find the biggest nerve plexus of the second brain, Auerbach's plexus (or the myenteric plexus). This innervates the muscles surrounding it and is responsible for gut movement during peristalsis. It extends up into the esophagus and down through the small intestine into the bowel.

Circular Muscle—Inner Layer of the Muscularis Externa

The next layer is the circular muscle that runs perpendicular to the longitudinal layer. They work together to create the strong wave-like motion required for gut function. Nerve fibers from Auerbach's plexus perforate this muscle and become finer to create the next layer.

Meissner's (Submucosal) Plexus

Meissner's plexus (or the submucosal plexus) is embedded in the submucosa, a dense irregular layer of connective tissue that supports the mucous membrane and connects it to the muscular layer. Fibers from the submucosal plexus reach through to the mucosa.

Mucosa

The mucosa is beneath the submucosa. The mucosa is made of several incredible layers: the lamina propria, the basement membrane, and the epithelial layer (which is next to the lumen, the hole in the middle, where we will reach the end of our journey).

Lamina Propria

The cell-rich lamina propria is a layer with loose tissue (I always picture a natural sponge), so there is room for many cells, including lymphocytes, enteric glial cells, neuroendocrine cells, mast cells, and immune cells. It also contains capillaries and lymph vessels. Its irregular surface allows it to connect well with the layers above and below. It provides support and nutrition to the epithelial layer and it has glands whose ducts open onto the mucosal epithelial layer next to the lumen. These glands secrete mucus and serous secretions.

Basement Membrane

We have now reached the basement membrane below the lamina propria and supporting the epithelial layer. The basement membrane is a thin, fibrous, extracellular matrix of tissue that separates the loose connective tissue of the lamina propria from the epithelial layer above. This kind of tissue is often considered to be fascia and, in my clinical experience, often holds tension and strain patterns.

Epithelial Layer

We have reached the epithelial layer and are nearly into the lumen—the space in the middle of the long tube. This thin epithelial tissue forms the outer layer of the body's innermost surface and lines the alimentary canal and other hollow structures. In the gut, it is a single layer of cells that covers all the nutrient-absorbing projections, called villi (fig. 5), that cover its surface. The epithelial layer is where absorption of nutrients takes place in the small intestine.

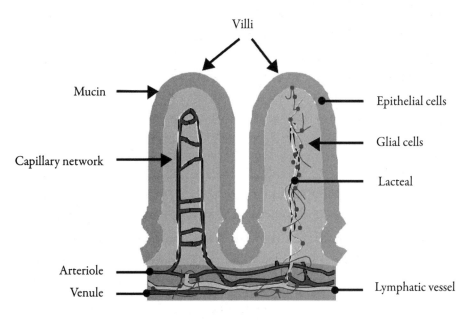

Figure 5. Cross section of intestinal villi.

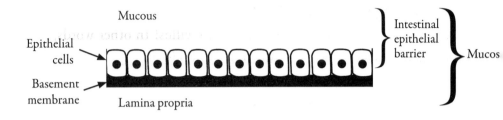

Figure 6. Intestinal epithelial barrier and mucosa.

The muscle contractions and the villi push the food through. There are no villi in the bowel (or large intestine), as we do not absorb many nutrients there. This single layer of epithelial cells creates the intestinal epithelial barrier that works hard to keep the bad guys out and let the good guys into our body (fig. 6). Epithelial cells are constantly being shed and replaced from the crypts in between the villi and only last for around four to five days. More about this will be shared later.

SMALL INTESTINE SURFACE AREA

To create as large a surface area as possible, three clever things happen here in the small intestine. First, the tube has tight, circular folds called the plicae circulares (visualize a slinky or hoover hose, or perhaps even a concertina). Second, villi—created by the mucosa pushing up into these waving projections—increase the surface area of the mucosa approximately sixtyfold. Third, microvilli cover the tip of nearly all the epithelial cells of the epithelial layer nearest the lumen (and do most of the absorbing of nutrients), thus increasing the absorptive surface approximately six-hundred-fold. These numerous microscopic microvilli (one hundred nanometers in diameter) form an undulating brush border.

Fascinating note: Enteric glia from the enteric nervous system reach through to the very tip of every single villus! In other words, our innermost layer touches what enters our body from the external environment. At this point, we are between two worlds. The outside world is coming into contact with our inside world.

To inspire you with wonder as we consider this place deep inside us, here is a poem I have written about the villi. I envision them as delicate tendrils reaching sensitively into the outside world as it comes inside.

Velvet Villi

Villi . . . microvilli
Thousands of delicate fingertips
Creating a velvet lining
Deep inside us

Touching our world inside
Absorbing the emotional rainbow
Of our daily lives

Fully charged with sparkling enteric glia
Scattered like stars in a night sky
In our inner universe

Pulsing networks of flashing calcium
As glia talk to neurons, cells and bacteria

All conversations shaped by
Feelings and experiences of generations past.

⬤ *Experience the Gut's Layers*

You might choose to take a few minutes to do the following exercise as a way to begin to care for your own gut.

The body loves to be listened to and touched. Keep that in mind as you lie down in a quiet place where you will not be disturbed, and place your hands gently on the lower part of your abdomen, where the small intestine and bowel are located. Take a few moments to relax and breathe deeply into that part of your body and into your hands.

Are your hands soft and comfortable? Notice how your body feels underneath them. Does it feel relaxed and warm? Perhaps it feels tense or tender? Maybe you feel nothing there, as if it is numb? There is no judgment here—just a curiosity and a desire to listen gently to the soft voice of the gut.

Use the outline below and write down your observations. You may feel tension in one layer and not in another; or you may have an emotional memory or just feel an emotion in another. Whatever you notice, make a note and see if that feeling changes as you stay there a few moments longer. You can always repeat this exercise another time and compare the experience.

Outline for Observations of the Gut's Layers

Skin

Superficial fascia just under the skin

Mesentery—connective tissue attaching to, enveloping, and suspending the small and large intestine from the back wall of the abdomen, carrying blood, nerve, and lymph supplies between the two layers

Longitudinal muscle

Auerbach's (or myenteric) nerve plexus

Circular muscle

Submucosal layer in which the smaller Meissner's (or submucosal) plexus is embedded

Lamina propria—full of cells of all kinds

Basement membrane

Villi—absorb nutrients and with enteric glia reach every tip

Epithelium

Lumen—internal space that is, in fact, the outside world coming into our body

Case Story—David
Listening to the Layers

David presented to me with severe long-term ulcerative colitis. He was in a lot of pain, was losing a lot of weight, and had severe diarrhea much of the time. His work as a consultant in the National Health Service was intense, and he was always under a large amount of pressure. He often worked six or seven days a week, but it was sometimes difficult for him to work as his energy levels were so low.

He had often been on steroids and did not like taking them. The next option would be surgery, which could potentially lead to the placement of a stoma.

We had a short initial session of thirty minutes. I began with my hands on his abdomen and simply listened to each of the different layers of the small intestine. I was soon focused on his basement membrane (remember: this supports the intestinal epithelial barrier). This presented to my hands with a strong pattern of tension and twisting. I stayed present with this layer and facilitated its unwinding and releasing. David became very relaxed and aware of the subtle movements and of the release in his abdomen.

Once this activity had settled down, I released his upper back (at the thoracic inlet, where the cervical spine in the neck meets the chunkier midspine or thoracic spine). Next, I released his occipital cranial base to release the environment around the all-important vagus nerve (which controls rest and digest).

These areas were all fairly restricted, and this was no surprise given the amount of work pressure he was under and the pain he had been in due to his gut problem. However, it all freed up, and he was nearly asleep. The next day, David sent me a message to say how much better he felt. His energy levels were better, his pain was diminished, and his gut was calmer.

We have continued to have short sessions whenever his work permits, and he has realized his working life needs to change in order to gain permanent improvement. David now plans to leave his current working role. He is already feeling more peaceful knowing that he has regained control of his life and that treatment can help his gut problems improve significantly.

This Story's Message

This case is a perfect illustration of how we never know where we might find tension and restriction in the layers of the intestine. In David's case, it was the basement membrane that was holding a lot of tension, which I unwound during his CranioSacral Therapy session. This was the area that came up in each treatment and release gave him huge relief from symptoms for at least two weeks afterward. Long-term changes occurred after he was able to adjust his work stress levels.

3
Searching for Stories in the Second Brain

Other memories are trying to get my attention now. "It wasn't just that cold, blue dive," they say. "We are where it all really began—talk to us." They are huddled like a group of homeless children in a doorway in a dark street somewhere. The street is somewhere inside my body. I feel compassion and sorrow as I glance at them. I walk toward them. I look at all their faces. Each one is so familiar to me now. Crouching with them in that doorway, I feel exposed. How to share a life that was far from perfect?

Memory: Skinny Baby

Nudging me is a memory holding a small, skinny baby in her arms, showing her to me. The baby is me just after I was born. Hovering behind us are the shadows of two men.

The memory of when I was conceived is possibly one of the only two times my mother shared honestly with me in a way that was a very small mitigation for all the rest of our shared journey on this earth. My mother told me that she and my father had been very fond of each other, and one day, they had lain naked in each other's arms amongst the tall grass by a river. This man was my biological father, whom I never met.

She told me this when I was seventeen, and I had just found out that my biological father was not her husband, Alfred, whom I had always seen as my father. It was very confusing. Alfred was the only family member who was not unkind to me, but he had no health or energy to do very much for me or with me. He was much older than my mother and always ill—tuberculosis, strokes, glaucoma. His life had become deeply unpleasant—he was unable to read due to his failing eyesight and married to a woman who was critical, disapproving, and unhappy herself. I remember him as confused, rising in the middle of the night to try to get me to put my school uniform on and go to school. Sitting in our living room silently with tears running down his face. He had nothing left to live for. He had set out with great potential and talent as an incredible singer, poet, writer, and teacher. All of these talents he explored, but as I was growing up, his world had been reduced to sitting for hours in silence and despair and wandering the house in confusion at night. I was filled with compassion for him.

My mother was desperate for attention in an unhappy marriage, and my biological father was unable to resist anything that would block out the pain of his own trauma. My mother was terrified that Alfred would find out that I was not his. I was conceived in a love between my mother and a man outside her marriage, but it was a love wrapped up in deceit and fear. I was born carrying my biological father's pain from his trauma. I was born into uncertainty and was the center of an ongoing lie.

Even at the beginning of my life I was caught between two worlds. I arrived not knowing how to eat, or perhaps not wanting to eat, as the outside world was already a frightening and overwhelming place. I could not digest any milk—or was it my mother's fear and anxiety I could not digest? A baby unsure of whether this world was a place I wanted to be in at all, I failed to thrive. Every day, the doctor came in despair to watch a baby, who did not want to be on this earth, slowly die.

Somewhere inside me, there must have been the strength to stay in this life, a will to survive. I eventually decided to accept the challenge of being in this world, and I suddenly and finally began to eat. I started to put on weight. Now I look back at how my digestion responded to the world outside and see that the stage was already set for what was to come.

Memory: Isolated Girl of Four

Another memory, quiet and downcast, steps into my mind now. She cannot look into my eyes. She is a little girl of four with brown hair and blue eyes, wearing a little blue smock dress, standing alone, intently watching children play at a nursery. I long to hold her in my arms. She is outside on a tarmac playground. In the middle is a big toy ship for climbing. I can see she would love to go and play on this ship. Other children at the nursery are already playing on it, scampering all over it, laughing, and making up stories. My heart skips a beat as I look at her. Her face is covered in loneliness, isolation, and anxiety. These feelings are creating a mask. Her light is dimmer already. Afraid of joining in and not being accepted, she stands always on the sidelines. It looks as if she doesn't know how to play with the other children, so she stays a little apart, watching, pretending she is okay.

But I can see that she is not okay. I wonder how no one else notices this. This gentle memory tiptoes often through my mind and has done so all my life. She wants to be seen and yet is equally afraid of being seen. I send this little girl so much love and compassion, and yet, she is still a little separate, a little wary of other people. These same feelings of separation and isolation still flow through me now and then.

Barrage of Memories

Other memories are coming thick and fast now out of that corner—shouting, tumbling, pushing, and shoving—making my heart sad and my head hurt with their noisy insistence. So much hitting, tears, confusion, loneliness, desperate sadness, criticism, lack of any connection between anyone in my life, lack of affection, lack of nurturing, lack of listening, and lack of encouragement—I cannot tell you any more for now. Perhaps I will later.

Memory: Fourteen Years Old, Tearless and Frozen

Wait, there is one more candidate just now, and I cannot ignore her. She is left alone in the corner, approaching me slowly when the others have given up, for now, and retreated. Her eyes are red and puffy from crying, and she is showing me a very still picture. I am around fourteen years old, maybe a little younger. The story did not change much over those years, so precision is not important. I am lying on my bed in my room. It is a large room with bay windows and a high ceiling. It is quite cold, as it is in an old Victorian house that has not been looked after very well. I spend a lot of time here. Many tears have fallen on the pillow while lying on my single bed, tucked behind the door. But this day I reach a point when I have no more tears. I remember this very clearly. I am listening to one of my favorite pieces of music, Faure's *Requiem Mass*. I am like a wave that cannot break. The tears won't come any more to bring even a temporary relief. I am caught in the tension of a sorrow that fills me but can no longer be expressed.

Perhaps it feels pointless to my body to keep crying. After all, no one comes to me, and nothing changes. I think that is important to note. I remember the tension in my stomach, in my whole abdomen. I remember the thick silence that falls around me as the tears stop. It is a silence that feels impossible to penetrate. It is a further separation. Imagine perhaps a wave, reaching its highest, most powerful moment, being frozen in time. I realize my body can still do that. I can separate, freeze, and be silent. It is not comfortable. This is the moment I learned how to do that.

I notice that when this happens, there is a stillness, and inside that stillness isn't peaceful. It is almost as if someone has pressed pause. It is suspension taking the place of feeling. Breathing almost stops. I am writing this wondering if this touches anyone else's experience. If it does, then you now know you are not alone. In fact, we probably have much to share. Just imagining you reading this, and feeling that someone else may have been in that dark place too, encourages me to continue a little longer.

I do not remember crying much after that day when I was fourteen. Perhaps I did but have forgotten. I remember many moments of sadness and shock after that time, but I can only see myself frozen. I did cry for several days a few years later when my first marriage fell apart. By then, I was twenty-three years old. At that time, I saw that I do not know how to be close to another person or to let someone into my world. I cried because of this discovery. It was devastating. But I am getting ahead of myself.

Memory: Ten-Year-Old with a Letter

There is another small group of quiet memories walking toward me from the shadows. These children are different ages, from around six to sixteen years old. They are wrapping the remnants of old clothes around them as they walk, all of them gray and streaked with dirt. Pulling these old clothes as tightly as they can around their shivering bodies, their eyes are empty and staring. I am wondering where these shadows are within me. I think they are in my gut.

I know what these memories are, but there was a time when I would have avoided them. These children are here to remind me of other times when I "froze." I saw them approaching earlier today, but I chose to look the other way. They did not react to my rejection; it is all too familiar for them. Perhaps I can see their eyes glaze over a little, retreat more deeply into a numb state as I turn away— that's all.

Why do I still walk away from them sometimes? After all the years I have been immersed in Upledger CranioSacral Therapy, together with all the work I have received, part of me still finds it hard to accept that these early experiences can affect my whole life in both positive and negative ways, that they are now part of me— integrated with the adult part of myself. Am I alone in this? Is it so surprising?

As children, we assume that the bad things that happen to us and around us are somehow our fault and that we are therefore not okay, not good enough, and are fundamentally flawed. If these events had happened to my children, I would be desperately sad for them and give them enormous amounts of support. But sometimes I struggle to apply the same approach to myself. There is more shame and confusion. Compassion for my younger self is not always easy to find, even now. Compassion and self-care have been learned gradually, and they are an ongoing process.

I invite one of these shadows to come forward, and this is what she tells me. I am about ten years old. I am in my mother's bedroom. (She and her husband Alfred had separate bedrooms all my life.) I am sitting at her dressing table, writing a note to my mother and Alfred, who, at that time, I still thought was my father. In the letter, I write that I do not believe they are my real parents. I suggest that somehow they must have taken me away from my real parents and adopted me. I feel desperate and alone, but I have no idea what happened before that moment. It is a complete blank, and that is interesting in itself. I wonder now what I thought would happen after they read this note. Perhaps in some part of my confused mind, I hoped they might return me to my real parents, who would be loving and kind. In my fantasy, these real parents are somewhere out there in the world and I believe if I can be reunited with them, I might feel like part of a family and feel less disconnected from everyone around me. I leave the note and go back to my own room, my body full of tension.

Later, my mother finds the note. I think she showed it to Alfred. They are *very* angry. I hear her running to my room, coming to find me, and my heart thumps. Even today, as I write this, my heart begins to beat faster and harder with fear. Red-faced and furious, she shouts at me that it was a terrible thing to say and that I am a horrible child. Even Alfred, her ailing husband, shouts at me. I don't remember any other time that he shouted at me.

I freeze. I do not apologize. I do not remember saying anything at all. What can I say? It is how I really feel.

She grabs me, drags me back into her bedroom, throws me down on her bed, and begins to hit me, over and over again, shouting at me. I am crying now and asking her to stop. When she has had enough, she storms out of the room and leaves me.

When she has gone, I come out of freeze into fight and flight. All my emotions explode. I am very angry and very hurt. I need to vent my anger. I pull on the curtains—hard—swinging on them, bending the curtain rails and ripping the fabric, until I have no strength left. I remember they were dark red velvet. I can still feel the soft velvet bunched up in my hands. I can see them hanging in tatters from the bent rails. I am shocked at how strong a very angry ten-year-old child can be. I return to my room.

When she finds the curtains, she shouts at me all over again, saying how bad I am. I cannot remember whether she hit me again. I spend the rest of the day in my room. My body returns to a numb, frozen state. It is as if every organ inside me is paused. I have learned how to be very, very quiet. I feel completely alone and helpless. My clumsy cry for some kind of help has completely misfired. My world is a dark and hopeless place that day.

I wonder what memories of this are carried in the cells of my gut. Writing this, I take a moment to listen to my inner world. I feel a slight vibration, almost a wobble, a sense of hiding and silence. As I connect with this, I feel sad and gather the young shadow memory up into my arms. Holding her is painful. The task feels overwhelming. We huddle together, she and I, arms around each other. Her body feels thin and contracted somehow. I wait for a warming, a softening. Perhaps it will take a while longer. I have all the time in the world for her. I have found compassion for my younger self.

Memory: Frozen Digestion

Peeping out from behind this still and dismal picture is another memory I cannot ignore. This one is looking a bit shamefaced at me. She is apologizing for coming forward but is reminding me that this book is about the gut. She is showing me that I often used to be constipated and take laxatives, that my digestion appears to have "frozen" too at times.

I was often constipated for many years, perhaps until my

early thirties, when I began my work on myself. Gradually my gut unfroze. As I began to have counseling and to live my own life, everything improved. I had not yet discovered Upledger CranioSacral Therapy.

My mother was severely constipated for most of her life and always took laxatives, right up until her death. She had Parkinson's disease for over ten years before her death, and, as I have discovered, this is often preceded by years of constipation. Perhaps she was in freeze in her gut? I don't know, and I wish I cared more. What I do know is that she could not express herself emotionally. The whole world was supposed to make her happy and make her life good, and when it didn't, it was someone else's fault. She was never an actor in her own life, only a reactor, bouncing from one emotional crisis and fantasy to the next, mostly unaware of the chaos she was creating all around her. I was always more her mother, albeit very reluctantly, than she mine. It was a burden that nearly broke me.

I was her maladjusted child. I received this diagnosis from a psychotherapist I saw several years ago. *Maladjusted* means unable to cope with the demands of a normal social environment—its connotations are disturbed, unstable, neurotic, alienated, muddled, and unbalanced. He was right. I was.

I feel sad sharing this. My gut must have been holding so many stories of violence, confusion, and grief. As I write, I feel some compassion for it, and for myself. This is a comparatively new feeling, which has taken a few years to create, and it is so welcome. I am now listening rather than judging—finally, or at least in this moment.

Today I am still fairly full of cold, not as fresh or clear as I would like to be. Apparently, that is still how it is meant to be. There is a tension high up in my stomach, which is very familiar across most of my life.

But any lowering of spirits following from this state of affairs is lifted right back up. I may have climbed out of bed with that wrecked, dried up, aching, cotton-wool-headed feeling you have with a cold; but when I looked out of the window, I saw bright clear sun, skies blue and yellow, with sharp white frost on the ground that made every fallen leaf speak of Christmas.

Remembering the glorious feeling invoked by this scene, I decide to take a pause from writing. Wrapping up very warmly, I head off for a gentle walk along the river to soak up the light and color, and breathe deep the cool, fresh air. A little way along the bank, I can see a group of people standing around, staring up at a tree. There is a black, rather scraggly-looking crow, stuck high up in the tree. Its feet are caught in some fishing wire among the tangled branches. Flapping helplessly, the crow cannot fly away. Someone called the Royal Society for the Prevention of Cruelty to Animals (RSPCA), but the RSPCA man is not allowed to climb trees. He called the fire brigade. The RSPCA man watches the fireman climbing the tree quietly and gently. The RSPCA man has a cage open and ready for the bird, which is lined with a comfortable pink blanket. I stand and watch the enormous care and skill the fireman and his team use to cut and pull the twisted, knotted tree branches out of the bird's way. It looks like a giant puzzle that they have to figure out, and they do. They manage to work out which branches to move and which to saw. Then, gently, with a rope, they pull down the branch with the now-panicking crow attached, all the way down, so the RSPCA man can reach it. The fireman first saws the piece of branch the exhausted bird is standing on to separate it from the rest. Then, the RSPCA man cuts the fishing wire extremely carefully from its feet and, holding the bird gently, places it in the comfortable cage. He'll take the bird to his clinic and check for injuries. The head fireman congratulates and thanks his men for a job well done. The RSPCA man thanks them, and the small crowd of bystanders applauds all four of the men. Everyone there cares about the life of one not-especially-beautiful black crow and works together, with compassion, to set it free. This beautiful illustration of love warms my heart and takes me forward into my life. Very few things in life are such a beautiful illustration of love. Perhaps this is the duality in all life—to see and feel the beauty and love we have and also to feel the fear, anger, and many other negative emotions. Or perhaps it is, as the inspiring Kahil Gibran said in *The Prophet:*

> *Your joy is your sorrow unmasked.*
> *And the selfsame well from which your laughter rises*
>   *was oftentimes filled with your tears.*
> *And how else can it be?*
> *The deeper that sorrow carves into your being, the*
>   *more joy you can contain.*
> *Is not the cup that holds your wine the very cup that*
>   *was burned in the potter's oven?*
> *And is not the lute that soothes your spirit, the very*
>   *wood that was hollowed with knives?*
> *When you are joyous, look deep into your heart and*
>   *you shall find it is only that which has given you*
>   *sorrow that is giving you joy.*
> *When you are sorrowful look again in your heart,*
>   *and you shall see that in truth you are weeping*
>   *for that which has been your delight.*

> *Some of you say, "Joy is greater than sorrow," and*
>   *others say, "Nay, sorrow is the greater."*

But I say unto you, they are inseparable.
Together they come, and when one sits alone with you
   at your board, remember that the other is asleep
   upon your bed.

Verily you are suspended like scales between your
   sorrow and your joy.
Only when you are empty are you at standstill and
   balanced.
When the treasure-keeper lifts you to weigh his gold
   and his silver, needs must your joy or your sorrow
   rise or fall.

This walk was created to lift and enliven. Returning along the path, I hear a soft symphony of crackles and pops, so I pause. On my left, a tree spreads its branches wide and low; its limbs are mostly bare now, with all the leaves gold and russet making a thick carpet underneath. I listen more carefully. Where are the instruments playing? What kind of elvish sound is this? At first, I wonder if it is the leaves crackling as they slowly warm in the sun, but then I see drops of melted frost falling from the branches in beautiful harmonies onto the crispy, white-edged leaves below, creating a secret natural musical score. Poetry fills my soul and gives me purpose again. These are the moments that allow me to expand into joy once more.

Today I needed that lifting up. My poor gut does not like the cold in my head, and I feel nauseous and weak. I would like to lie down and curl up. But if I did that every time I felt like this, I would do nothing in my life since I have felt like this often. So, instead, I sit here after my walk, a little slumped now, and talk to you.

✳

I have committed to describing my journey through this book, and I hope you can use my story to begin yours. Here is how you can begin.

Recall that in the appendix of the book is a page that prompts you: "If your gut could make a face right now, what would it look like?" Take a moment to listen to your digestive tract and see how it feels. What kind of face would it make? Without thinking too hard, just draw whatever pops up in your awareness. You don't need to be an artist, just draw any image you see.

Why drawing? Because it is a way of both avoiding and sneaking under our rational, always-ready-to-judge, self-censoring part of our mind that is so good at covering up the deeper stories we hold inside us. If you find this is a helpful way to stay more connected with this part of yourself, you might like to do this on a daily basis and perhaps make notes based on the expression you find yourself drawing. Perhaps write down what you have just eaten, or what was going on for you emotionally at the time, or what you were doing that day. If you want something beyond a notebook of blank pages, you can also purchase my tummy tracker journals at the Upledger Institute's website and the International Alliance of Healthcare Educators' website.

Case Story—Baby Oliver
Tension and Release

Baby Oliver came to me at seven weeks old with colic—in other words, problems with wind and anxiety. After feeding, especially in the evenings, he found it very difficult to release gas, and it was becoming trapped lower in his system. Oliver would become very upset, and his parents found it almost impossible to soothe him or help him settle.

Oliver had a difficult birth, as he was helped out with forceps after becoming stuck in the birth canal, leaving bruising to his face around the cheekbones.

He laid on my couch, curled up around his belly, grimacing and crying. My hands-on evaluation showed me there was a large amount of tension in the abdomen and also around the top of the neck, the cranial base.

I began with my hands, working on the lower part of his spine and belly, listening to and following patterns of tension in his intestines to begin facilitating release. He began to uncurl and relax a little. Part of this process was a lot of farting, which caused some welcome laughter in the treatment room! During the releasing process, he would sometimes look agitated and anxious and cry a little before settling again. This was very likely a release of the emotions he might have felt during his birth experience. As a small baby, the only way he could express these was through crying. This is how babies tell us their stories.

Next I gently released his neck and occipital cranial base (the place where the skull sits on the top of the spine), then very lightly contacted his sphenoid (a butterfly-shaped cranial bone that runs across the skull behind the eyes and forms part of the floor of the cranium), decompressing it and aligning it. My attention was taken to the pituitary gland (this sits in the sphenoid and sparks the whole endocrine [hormone] system and is often involved in the stress and upset of colicky babies). The occipital cranial base release also creates a healthy environment for the passage of the vagus nerve into the body, which is a huge part of a healthy digestive process. His whole body relaxed, and he went from being a curled-up ball of unhappiness to a contented starfish lying on his back, arms and legs spread out. His parents were surprised and delighted.

This Story's Message

Babies often come for treatment after a mother's difficult pregnancy or birth, or both, which leaves tension and misalignment in the baby's body. These tension patterns are often found in the dural membrane that lines the cranium (skull) and at the top of the neck where the skull meets the top of the spine at the first cervical vertebra. The mother's emotional status during her pregnancy may also play a part in the level of tension in the growing fetus. I am quite sure I was born with a high level of tension around my nervous system due to my mother's high stress and fear levels.

4

Finding Compassion for Your Gut's History

ADVERSE CHILDHOOD EXPERIENCES

Early emotional experiences have a lasting impact on lifelong mental and physical health. The root of the disturbance occurs in the gut. The Adverse Childhood Experience (ACE) Study[4] is a research study conducted by the American health care company Kaiser Permanente and the Centers for Disease Control and Prevention. A total of seventeen thousand participants were recruited between 1995 and 1997 and have been in long-term follow-up for health outcomes. The study has been analyzed extensively and is frequently cited as a notable landmark in epidemiological research. The study has produced more than fifty scientific articles and more than one hundred conference and workshop presentations that look at the prevalence and consequences of adverse childhood experiences.

The study demonstrated an association between adverse childhood experiences and health and social problems as an adult. One startling and central discovery was made: the most significant contribution to your lifelong health—both physical and mental—is your childhood experience. Childhood trauma affects your whole life. It changes the way your brain grows: you develop fewer circuits in your hippocampus for processing things and have more ready-to-go circuits in your amygdala that build anxiety and overreaction, hypervigilance, and fear. Childhood trauma also leaves memories in cells throughout your body and molecular footprints in the sand of your body's tissues. Your gut bacteria are influenced in a number of ways as well. At birth, the gut is colonized immediately from the birth canal of the mother and thereafter from skin contact, such as from the lips of the mother when she kisses her child. If the baby is born via C-section, if a baby has a difficult birth, if the mother has had a difficult pregnancy emotionally and/or physically, or if the baby is put in an incubator or high dependency unit, then the gut bacteria population will be diminished and less diverse. These babies may then have "leaky guts" as a result, and fewer bacteria will be present in the mucus of the lining of the intestines to protect the baby from bad bacteria.

Early physical and emotional attachment to their mother is very important to create enough healthy gut bacteria. Meaning, babies separated from mum in the first week or more, for medical or other reasons, will have all the above negative impacts on their gut bacteria as well as the above-mentioned issues with brain development and the digestive tract as a whole. If the mother is not able to be there, skin to skin time with either the father or another consistent caregiver (and most of all having a consistent, loving caregiver) will provide the early emotional and physical attachment needed to create safety and good development.

Studies of early years' trauma show that it affects the gut-brain axis; the gut microbiome; the sensory nerves in the digestive tube, which become oversensitive to normal sensations as a result; and the flow of blood to the intestines, which early years' trauma reduces.

There will be inflammation in the gut, which is associated with lack of diversity in gut bacteria and can lead to our bodies making antibodies that attack us. This is what happens when a person develops an autoimmune disease. Chronic stress, trauma, and physical as well as emotional attachment trauma therefore impacts the gut bacteria, which are always working with and talking to the enteric nervous system and the intestinal epithelial barrier. Due to adverse experience, the microbiome and enteric nervous system create inflammation states and potentially begin the process of autoimmune disease. One important point is that these changes in the gut-brain axis and microbiome do not automatically revert to a healthier state once the trauma is over. This is where doing our emotional work is important, especially through the SomatoEmotional Release process of CranioSacral Therapy.

Having had adverse childhood experiences that impact the second brain and the brain in the head, we see and respond to our whole life with these two brains that have been influenced by our early experiences. Our personality, our behavior, our ability to connect with others, and our ability to develop as individuals are all adversely affected, as are our self-image and beliefs.

How these early traumas affect the development and structure of the second brain and the microbiota is a vibrant research area, and there is much to learn. This discussion of the impact of adverse childhood experience on us throughout our lives leads us to our next topic, neuroplasticity, which gives us reason to hope for the possibility of change, integration of these experiences, and a happier future.

NEUROPLASTICITY

Norman Doidge was at the front of a raft of neuroscientists who brought us the incredible discovery of neuroplasticity in his book

The Brain that Changes Itself.[5] Neuroplasticity is now an accepted characteristic of the brain.

Neuroplasticity researchers explain that the brain is always changing and adapting to our environment and the information coming in through all our senses. Eighty percent of the activity of our brain is processing the sensory information coming in through proprioception, sight, hearing, touch, taste, smell, and interoception (our felt sense of our inner world). All our senses are interconnected and interdependent, and ideally all this information needs to be integrated well, so that we can decide what to do and what action to take or not take. How we process this information is influenced by our history, including our beliefs about ourselves and the world as a result of our experience. Doing so is a continuous interactive process between our central nervous system and the outside world. It is a work in progress our whole life.

If we have certain thought patterns about life, our brain will have pathways and synapses strongly wired for those patterns, like a well-trodden path through a forest. To make a new path, which might be more helpful to us in terms of our thinking or acting, we have to make an effort to tread that new path many times before it is easy to find and to walk. This is the essence of neuroplasticity. After trauma, whether that trauma is emotional or physical, such as a stroke, the brain can make new synapses with the right regular input; it can make new pathways, and we can learn to respond differently to the world; we can learn to walk again or talk again or use our arms again. We now recognize that neuroplasticity enables us to approach working with the brain in a very positive and hopeful way, knowing that the brain is capable of rewiring or changing. This is all good news, as we see how our brain is always fluid and adaptable and that it responds to input from external and internal influences. The new insights and research into the enteric nervous system would suggest this. This is a message of hope and possibility that opens to us infinite potential for change and healing.

Glial Cells

Just as exciting as the discovery of neuroplasticity is the discovery that glial cells play a part in the plasticity of neurons and that our neurons cannot exist without glial cells. Through our increasing understanding over the last fifteen years or so, we have learned much about the role of these little cells in our central and peripheral nervous system, including how they help us have a healthy nervous system and how they support our neuroplasticity. It turns out the glial cells are also the guardians of memory and learning and are a huge part of our creativity. In addition:

- They take care of and surround every neuron and every synapse between neurons.
- They regulate neuronal activity.
- They talk to each other in waves of calcium signaling (a series of molecular and biophysical events that link an external stimulus to the expression of an intracellular response; this is different from the more linear communication of neurons via synapses).
- They make the myelin sheathing that surrounds the axons to provide efficient and speedy communication between neurons.
- They are the brain's own immune system, rushing to the site of any infection or brain injury.
- They provide a convection system, called the glymphatic system, to take cerebrospinal fluid through the brain tissue, where it can supply nutrients and carry away unwanted proteins. If these proteins, especially amyloid beta proteins, stack

up and stay in our tissue, we are more likely to develop some kind of dementia or Alzheimer's. In addition, the demise of glial cells is beginning to be implicated in many kinds of disease and neurological dysfunction.

As CranioSacral therapists, we can use this new knowledge and awareness, as well as new techniques, when we are working on the nervous system of the person on the table, and by doing so we can have a more positive impact on their health.

Glial cells are smaller than neurons and outnumber them in the brain by at least six to one, perhaps ten to one. They were thought for many years to act solely as the glue that holds the neurons together in order to provide a matrix to support the brain tissue. But with new imaging techniques, we have discovered a whole new world that is highly relevant to Upledger CranioSacral therapists, allowing us to better assist the people who come to us. Indeed, the updated imagery is significant to anyone interested in their brain and spinal cord health.

What made Einstein so clever and so creative was that his brain contained many more glial cells than most other human beings.[6]

To find out everything you always wanted to know about glial cells but were afraid to ask, read *Brain Stars: Glial Cells Illuminating CranioSacral Therapy,* the book of my colleague and fellow Upledger Instructor Tad Wanveer.[7] To read about dementia and aging and CranioSacral Therapy, I direct you to another colleague and Upledger Instructor, Michael Morgan, and his book *The Body Energy Longevity Prescription: How CranioSacral Therapy Helps Prevent Alzheimer's and Dementia While Improving the Quality of Your Life.*[8]

ENTERIC NERVOUS SYSTEM PLASTICITY

Now that we know that the brain has plasticity, and we know the cells in part responsible for the plasticity, we must ask ourselves: Is there also plasticity in the second brain, the enteric nervous system that innervates most of the long tube from our mouth to our anus? It is full of enteric neurons and enteric glial cells like those responsible for neuroplasticity in the brain, so we can begin to imagine the impact of this. There is less research to date on enteric glia, but they are turning out to be just as important in the second brain as in the first brain. If I have whetted your appetite for more, read about both brains in the later chapter, "Peering down the Microscope."

Much of this enteric nervous system can make its own decisions as well as send messages via the vagus nerve up to our brain in the head. Many more messages are sent from the brain in our gut, our second brain, to the brain in our head, than the other way around. We have seen that the enteric nervous system is a large and vibrant data processing center. Is it so strange to wonder whether we have neuroplasticity and glial plasticity in the second brain too? This would open up infinite possibilities for healing and change in the enteric nervous system and the digestive system as a whole.

Neuroplasticity and glial plasticity in the enteric nervous system supports the idea that the second brain and gut are influenced and molded by our experiences from conception onward, and back through generations. These experiences might be emotional, physical, chemical, environmental, or any combination of these.

IMPACT OF CHILDHOOD TRAUMA ON THE GUT AND AUTONOMIC NERVOUS SYSTEM

If early trauma impacts brain development in the head, surely it will also impact the brain in your gut and the microbiota. In fact, a study by gastroenterologist Emeran A. Mayer and researchers titled "Differences in Gut Microbial Composition Correlate with Regional Brain Volumes in Irritable Bowel Syndrome"[9] showed that people with early life trauma have a different microbiome from those without.

As we have seen, our gut and our brain develop and grow according to all our experiences. Thus early life trauma can also have long-term impacts on your autonomic nervous system. It may leave your autonomic nervous system tuned to fight, flight, or freeze as its default state.

At this point it might be helpful to pause and look at our autonomic nervous system. This system takes care of our breathing, eating, sleeping, and other automatic functions without our having to think about them, so that we can do more advanced stuff like work, play sports, play music, talk to friends, and so on. The traditional concept is that the autonomic nervous system has two branches.

- The **sympathetic** nervous system is our fight and flight system that opens our airways and sends blood to our muscles so that we can fight or run away from a threatening or dangerous situation.
- The **parasympathetic** nervous system manages our ability to rest, switch off, store energy, and digest our food when we feel safe.

The sympathetic system is a high consumer of energy, whereas the parasympathetic system is a conserver of our energy with a slower metabolic burn.

POLYVAGAL THEORY

Over the last ten years or so, knowledge of the enteric nervous system and the autonomic nervous system has expanded. Stephen Porges's polyvagal theory[10] leads us into a more complex grasp of our autonomic nervous system and our vagus nerve in particular, and this more complex understanding influences our comprehension of the enteric nervous system. In turn, this new knowledge of the vagus nerve and enteric nervous system affects our cognizance of resilience, well-being, child development, and many other areas.

Stephen Porges reveals that there are two branches of the vagus nerve that arise from separate ganglions* in the brain stem: the ventral vagal complex and the dorsal vagal complex. They differ from each other in function and purpose.

He suggests the dorsal vagal complex is the oldest part of the vagal system† and is mostly located from our respiratory diaphragm downward into our abdomen. It is concerned with and connected to our gut, our breathing, and our digestion. It is also strongly connected to our enteric nervous system.

Porges suggests that our ventral vagal complex has evolved comparatively more recently than the dorsal vagal complex. The ventral vagal complex helps facilitate all our facial expressions, head turning

---

*A ganglion is a mass of nerve tissue containing nerve cells where signals from nerves enter and exit.
†The vagal system includes the ventral vagus nerve and the dorsal vagus nerve.

and tilting mechanisms, eye contact, voice tone, and everything involved in connecting with another human being or animal. In other words, the ventral vagal complex is all about social engagement, attachment, and feeling safe. The ventral vagal complex is found above the respiratory diaphragm.

The way the enteric nervous system fits into polyvagal theory is a brand new area of research, and the role of the enteric nervous system in polyvagal theory is yet to be thoroughly understood. The enteric nervous system is mostly below the respiratory diaphragm and is connected strongly to the dorsal vagal complex, the oldest part of our vagus nerve. When we feel afraid and go past our fight and flight instincts—into freeze, shutdown, disconnection, and disassociation—it is because of our dorsal vagal complex, and our gut, our enteric nervous system, is impacted.

A recent study titled "The Early Development of the Autonomic Nervous System Provides a Neural Platform for Social Behavior: A Polyvagal Perspective"[11] gives us the neurobiological mechanisms through which a newborn infant develops and matures their autonomic nervous system and how that is influenced by their interaction with their primary caregiver. This is where it becomes especially interesting and relevant to our exploration of the gut and early trauma. A baby's nervous system will model itself on input from the surrounding adults, especially the mother or primary caregiver. Our ventral vagal complex (the one concerned with social interaction and attachment) only works well if it is developed by our mother or primary caregiver at an early age, and this will only happen if the mother's or primary caregiver's ventral vagal complex is well tuned. A mother who is able to make healthy attachments and interact with people close to her will make a healthy, close attachment to her baby. She will mirror the baby's expressions, talk to her baby, repeat and mirror the sounds the baby makes, use a calm and playful tone of voice, and pick up and cuddle the baby. She will be calm (most of the time) and not in fight, flight, or freeze. If the mother were to be in one of those autonomic states, she would not be able to engage with her baby in a way that helps to promote the healthy development of the ventral vagal complex. Rather she might be angry, withdrawn, or distant. In these situations, the baby would become upset, lack the stimulation and growing attachment to their mother, or perhaps feel scared or alone. The baby might go into their own fight, flight, or even freeze.

The more we are in one autonomic state—fight, flight, or freeze—the more our autonomic nervous system will be accustomed to being in that state. It will either remain in it or go into it very easily and quickly. It becomes our default state. The usual or default state of the nervous system of a baby's primary caregiver will create a default to which the baby becomes tuned. The actions of social engagement and attachment are facilitated by the ventral vagal complex (e.g., facial expression, head tilting, hand and arm gestures, etc.). The baby will develop this part of their autonomic nervous system through practice and it will become a default state for the baby.

This process actually begins even before birth in the womb. Imagine a pregnant woman who is experiencing intense negative emotions, such as fear, guilt, or anger. How will this impact her baby? Compare this with a mother who is happy, content, and looking forward to the birth of her child. Imagine the difference in the levels of cortisol in each mother, the amount of tension in the fascia in each mother, the sound of her voice that reaches her unborn child, and the bacteria in her gut. Each mother's emotional state and the default state of her nervous system (which is perhaps normally in fight or flight) also reaches the child. How will the baby in utero experience all this? How will a mother's fight or flight state impact the development of the baby's brain and second brain and eventually its microbiome?

Imagine a mother with a lack of social skills, a lack of emotional intelligence—whose own central nervous system and autonomic nervous system are already set to a default of fight, flight, or freeze. Her baby's central and enteric nervous systems will likely already be molded by his or her in utero experience. Once the baby is born, he or she will then learn from the mother's emotional responses how to connect in only this way with the people that come into his or her life, or perhaps will learn not to connect at all. This mother will not be able to tune and develop her baby's nervous systems into a balanced, stable state.

This is yet another example of how difficult experiences are passed down through the generations. It seems likely that the enteric nervous system, our second brain, is neuro- and glial-plastic. We know it responds to our emotions and experiences. It receives messages from the vagus nerve as well as thinks for itself. Is it so far-fetched to wonder if this part of our nervous system is tuned by our mother or primary caregiver, just as the rest of our autonomic nervous system is? I wonder, therefore, if the structure of our enteric nervous system is influenced by our experiences in the womb and after birth while we are young. How does this system respond to lack of affection or attention or touch? If we do not feel safe when young, what impact does that have on our second brain? It is through healthy, early tuning of all these systems that we build our resilience to stress and develop our ability to digest food and sleep well. Have a look at my new model of the different strands of our autonomic nervous system, and notice that the enteric nervous system is included as one of its branches.

NEW MODEL OF THE AUTONOMIC NERVOUS SYSTEM

The second brain in the gut is the enteric nervous system and microbiota. It is part of the autonomic nervous system and it is closely involved with our fight and flight / rest and digest responses to our life experiences. It receives the outside world inside us.

Dorsal Vagal Complex/ Parasympathetic	Sympathetic Nervous System	Ventral Vagal Complex/ Parasympathetic	Enteric Nervous System
Large primitive nerve Common to all animals including fish Moderates heart rate Aids digestion When not in freeze, supports sleep, relaxation, meditation Responds to gentle touch, connection	Exercise Exertion Emotional/ sexual arousal Stress	Recent addition to mammals that need to raise children Influences muscles of face, expression, eye contact Functions when a person feels safe Attachment/social behavior is a way to avoid or come out of fight or flight	Connects with vagal complex Actively involved in flight or fight and freeze responses Autonomous aspect is our second brain
Freeze Occurs when sympathetic is too aroused and fight or flight are not working Shuts down whole system Associated with trauma and shame	Fight or Flight Spikes during moments of severe stress/ arousal		

⟶ Transition path

⟶ Influence/triggers

The nervous system in all its complexity in the body is like an embroidered fabric: threads from the vagus nerve and from polyvagal theory, threads from the enteric glia and their role in the enteric nervous system, and the threads of understanding how our earlier experiences shape our enteric nervous system create a more dynamic picture of the tapestry that is our nervous system. These threads tune the body to a particular frequency, setting us up for how we might respond to events that are challenging later in life. The new threads here are bringing the enteric nervous system into this tapestry and looking at how polyvagal theory can expand our understanding of how the enteric nervous system is influenced by our lives.

RESEARCH INTO PHYSIOLOGICAL CONNECTIONS BETWEEN GENERATIONS

I have been talking about one generation, but when a woman is pregnant with a daughter, the daughter already has all the eggs she will ever have in her ovaries. In this situation, we have three generations already connected. Multigenerational connections are being talked about in many ways now. Some suggest that children and grandchildren of Holocaust survivors are more predisposed to depression and anxiety as a result of what happened to their parents or grandparents.[12] Further studies in the following paragraphs show physiological connections between generations.

Aversions Passed through Two Generations

Studies on mice show how negative experiences and trauma can be passed down. Researchers gave a group of mice small electric shocks while at the same time giving the mice cherry blossoms to smell. As a result, the mice developed an aversion to that smell. The researchers found that the offspring of the mice also did not like the smell of cherry blossoms, even though they were not part of the experiment.[13] This aversion to the scent has been passed through two generations.

New studies in the field of epigenetics show that some individual tags* on genes remain through conception and are not all cleaned off during the fertilization process, as was originally thought.[14] This means that epigenetic changes can be passed on to the next generation. This study is part of the emerging science on how trauma may be passed on a neurobiological level through the generations.

MicroRNA Disruption through Three Generations

Hereditary trauma has long been known in psychology. Now its physiological basis is becoming known. "There are diseases such as bipolar disorder, that run through families but cannot be traced back to a particular gene," explains Isabelle Mansuy, professor at ETH Zurich.[15] With her research group at the Brain Research Institute, University of Zurich, she has been studying the molecular processes involved in nongenetic inheritance of behavioral symptoms induced by traumatic experiences in early life.

Mansuy and her team identified an important component of short RNA molecular processes. These RNAs, called microRNAs, are involved in the regulation of gene expression.

The researchers studied the number and kind of microRNAs produced by adult mice that they exposed to traumatic conditions in early life. When compared with corresponding cells of control animals, they discovered that traumatic stress alters the amount of several microRNAs in the blood, brain, and sperm, respectively; while there were too many of some microRNAs, there were too few of others. These alterations upset the regulation of cellular processes that the microRNAs would normally control.

---

*Gene tags are the short sequences of proteins that result in a person's unique genetic expression.

After traumatic experiences, the mice behaved differently—they lost their natural dislike of open spaces and bright light and became depressed. These changes were passed to the next generation via sperm, even though the offspring were not exposed to any traumatic stress themselves.

The metabolism of the children of stressed mice was also negatively affected—their insulin and blood sugar levels were lower than in children of nontraumatized parents. "We were able to demonstrate for the first time that these changes are hereditary," says Mansuy. The effects on metabolism and behavior carried on to the third generation.

"With the imbalance in microRNAs in sperm, we have discovered a key factor through which trauma can be passed on," explains Mansuy. However, there remains the question of how the dysregulation in short RNAs happens. Mansuy continues, "Most likely, it is part of a chain of events that begins with the body producing too many stress hormones."

Mansuy and her team are now studying the role of short RNAs in human inheritance of trauma.

Information Passed through Fourteen Generations

A team led by scientists from the European Molecular Biology Organization (EMBO) in Spain studied genetically engineered nematode worms that carry a transgene for a fluorescent protein. This gene made the worms glow when put under ultraviolet light. When the researchers changed the temperature of the worms' containers, worms kept at twenty degrees Celsius showed low activity of the transgene; the worms hardly glowed at all. But when they moved the worms to a warmer temperature of twenty-five degrees Celsius, the worms suddenly lit up like little wormy Christmas trees! This meant the fluorescence gene had become much more active. When the worms were moved back to cooler temperatures, the worms continued to glow brightly, suggesting they were holding on to an environmental memory of the warmer climate and that the transgene was still highly active.

Furthermore, that memory was handed down to their offspring for a whole seven brightly glowing generations. None of these offspring had ever experienced the warmer temperatures. The baby worms inherited this epigenetic change through both eggs and sperm.

The team then pushed the results even further. They kept five generations of worms at twenty-five degrees Celsius and then put their offspring in colder temperatures. They watched to see what would happen. Astonishingly, the worms continued to have higher transgene activity. By the end of the experiment, they glowed more brightly for an unprecedented fourteen generations.[16]

That is the longest scientists have ever observed the passing down of an environmentally induced genetic change. The scientists wondered if this was a kind of biological planning ahead for survival of the species. By predicting what their environment might be like in the future, they enabled their descendants to better survive.

Inherited Trauma without Changing DNA

Inherited effects like these in humans are difficult to measure because we live a lot longer than worms. But research carried out by Uppsala University of Finland in conjunction with the National Institutes of Health and the University of Helsinki, published under the title "Association of the World War II Finnish Evacuation of Children with Psychiatric Hospitalization in the Next Generation," does imply that events in our lives can affect the development of our children.[17]

✳

The studies referred to above begin to illuminate the potential impact of the personal and environmental experiences of previous generations on each of us, on our children, and on our grandchildren. While these studies are not directly about the gut, we know the gut is the root of much mental and physical ill health, that it has its own memory systems, that it is intimately connected with our autonomic and central nervous system, that the microbiome has its own set of genes that we are beginning to study, and that early life trauma has a major impact on its health. I hope that all this will expand your view of the potential influences on your gut and any issues you have with it in an empowering way. There is so much we do not know yet.

Biological Father, Kostek

In addition to being influenced by my mother, I know that my gut has also been influenced by at least one other person—my father. I know that my gut has also been influenced by at least one generation ahead of me.

My biological father, Kostek, was from a part of Poland that was sometimes in the Ukraine, depending on where the border was at any given time. He was a brave man and was awarded the Virtuti Militari (the Polish equivalent of the Victoria Cross) as well as the Cross of Valour four times for various courageous acts in the face of the enemy, including bringing a wounded bomber plane home. He fled his country after watching all his family massacred in front of his eyes. This trauma marked him for the rest of his life.

He came to the United Kingdom as a refugee and flew as a navigator in the Air Force until the end of the war. Once settled here in the United Kingdom, he ran a successful import-export business and became a highly respected bronze sculptor.

One of the small insights my mother gave me was that he asked her not to judge his people by the ones who fled to the United Kingdom. He told her that they were changed by what they had seen. I believe he drank quite a lot and probably, although he had an English wife and children, had affairs with more women than just my mother.

But I have no feeling of judgment or blame for him. I have compassion for him, since he witnessed his family's violent deaths. Would it be so surprising, in the light of the above research, that he passed some of his experience on to me? In fact, I think it would be more surprising if he had not. His genes would have been tagged and then those tags passed on to me. Some of my emotional pain is probably his—passed on. It feels like there is still some pain held in my digestive tract somewhere. Being aware of this and sending him love and compassion seems to help me. It took many years to be able to think of him with love rather than anger or hurt at what I perceived to be his rejection of me.

Case Story—Sheila
Overcoming the Effects of Trauma
on Our Gut and Mind

Sheila was a lady in her sixties who came to see me for problems with her bowels. Diagnosed with irritable bowel syndrome, her bowel movements were so loose, frequent, and urgent that she could not leave the house or consider going out without taking codeine to slow down her bowels' activity. The codeine was prescribed to her by her doctor. This was having a huge impact on her energy levels, and on her ability to live and enjoy her life fully. She came to see if I could help.

I would spend much of our sessions working on what I thought, at that time, was her pelvic diaphragm in order to release tension and rebalance it. I was probably palpating tension patterns in various layers in her intestines.

After a few sessions, her bowel had calmed considerably. As she became aware of the need for her own emotional release in order to release the emotional struggles of her parents and was able to express this, the layers of her gut were able to let go and the tissue memory, or cell memory, was released. Gradually the hypersensitivity of the gut reduced. She was able to go out without taking codeine and began to regain confidence in her bowel.

Sheila moved away at this point in her story, so I don't know how long this state lasted or whether she was able to get someone in her new area to help her and give her treatments when necessary. I hope so. After all, life keeps happening to us, and in turn our body. When we are under stress and challenges, our body can begin to revert to old patterns. It pays to recognize this and keep listening to, supporting, and nurturing our body-mind system in whatever ways work best for us, without waiting for uncomfortable symptoms to return or appear.

I am using the term body-mind *because they are one and the same. You cannot talk about the body without talking about the mind and vice versa. Dr. John E. Upledger said to those who were skeptical about the unity of the body and mind, "Show me where the body ends and the mind begins."*

This Story's Message

Sheila's story illustrates how trauma can be passed on through the generations and impact the reactivity of our bowels. It seemed that the trauma of her parents was passed on to her, possibly on many levels, the epigenetic and autonomic level being two of them. It also demonstrates that the effects of this trauma on the body and mind can be overcome with effort.

5
Container for Shame

The Tea Party Memory

Another memory, shamefaced, is standing somewhere far away with her back to me. Slowly she turns around and comes a little closer. She cannot look me in the eye and shuffles around the edges of my awareness. Eventually she crouches in a corner with her head in her hands. As I think of her now, sitting here writing to you, I can feel a familiar urge to avoid her story, a heaviness in my chest, and an echo of this memory falling like a stone into my gut. But I don't turn away because I am committed to sharing my story with you. I sit down beside her and hold one of her hands. Small, cold fingers weave into my fingers, and as our palms touch, I feel the fear in this holding. Also, I sense a desire for reassurance. This makes me feel very sad, and I wish I had held her hand a long time ago.

The memory tells me her story. I was nine years old, a little girl dressed in a frock and a cardigan, with bobbed brown hair and blue-gray eyes. Some innocence and hope was still left in that young face among the confusion.

I was sitting around a table where my mother and I were having tea. We were in her bungalow. My mother's colleague, Pete, was there, there were other people there too, and Pete's mother was there.

There must have been about eight people sitting around a big table covered in a tea service, sandwiches, and cakes. I didn't know who they were. I think I already suspected that my mother and Peter were becoming more than just friends—perhaps they already were. Alfred, my mother's husband at that time, was not there.

I cannot remember anything I said; in fact, I don't remember talking at all, as I felt so withdrawn from other people, but I must have said something that my mother did not like. Perhaps I made a comment about her and Pete, suggesting they were in a hidden relationship; I don't know. Whatever it was, my mother turned on me in front of everyone, red-faced and full of anger, and slapped me hard across my face. It hurt a great deal. She did not apologize to me or to any of the other guests for that matter. The imprint of her hand was clearly on my face for the rest of the day. Everyone was shocked. No one spoke. I froze and did not do anything. I did not say anything. She did not touch me again. She did not smile at me. The rest of that tea party has disappeared from my memory.

I do remember sitting very still, with my mother's handprint on my face and my cheek red and smarting. I looked down at my lap and did not meet anyone's eyes. I felt embarrassed and ashamed, feelings that were becoming quite familiar to me. I wanted to disappear. When we returned home, that incident was never referred to again. That is how it was during my childhood and teenage years: a conspiracy of silence, with everything buried under the surface. Nothing is understood or discussed, and feelings and emotions are most definitely never shared. I feel sick as I share this with you, and felt sick at the time, as yet another layer was added to the challenges my gut would face.

I learned from the beginning not to share my feelings and that sharing my feelings is not okay. I had no role models who could show me how this could be done in a mature way. The only times emotions leaked out in our house was through accusations and name calling, and through anger, violence, and sorrow.

Whenever my mother needed someone to lie for her to Alfred, my "father," I was the first person she asked. In my teenage years, the man I thought was my father became increasingly old and ill, and I know my mother was seeing Pete behind his back. This is in spite of the fact that Pete visited the house as a "friend." I never liked him. I always felt there was a sleaziness and sliminess about him. I hated it when he touched me, which it felt like he did too often. All my interactions with him left me feeling a little dirty. When my mother had a tryst with Pete, she told, not asked, me to lie to Alfred about where she was. A meeting of some sort was usually the excuse I was to offer him. She never told him anything herself, just disappeared out into the night. I had no way of resisting this. If I were to say anything, I would be beaten. Inevitably, she went out, and when Alfred, sitting silently by the fire in the evening, would ask me where she had gone, I would lie for her and say she was at a meeting. I hated doing this. I saw his sadness, and I saw that he knew it was not true. He probably knew I had no choice as well. We played this tragic pantomime over and over again. It slowly broke my heart. His was already broken. I was deeply ashamed.

Father Sings

But wait, suddenly and surprisingly, there is one beautiful memory now standing in front of me. She just appeared, expanding in front of me. She is singing to me. Her voice is wobbly, but the tone is clear and full of her own distant memories. Her song is a joyful, hopeful pause among all this despair, a signpost for my future. It comes to me from a long way away and takes me to another place. It is wonderful to sometimes travel to another, distant place, even if only for a few minutes. Have you ever experienced this? This is what the arts have always done for me. Whether through dance, theater, music, or poetry, the arts have helped me transcend reality and travel to another realm. Here emotions are accepted, understood, and resonate, if I am lucky, with those in the picture, piece of music, or the dance. In that moment, I am not alone. There, I feel connected and perhaps even hopeful.

I want to listen to this beautiful child singing. What message has she brought to me?

My family is sitting at the table one Sunday at lunchtime—my mother, Alfred, and me. For a short while that day, my mother was not screaming at him, and he was not returning her abuse. I do not remember how this happened or what led up to it, but Alfred began to sing. His voice was deep and full. It was shaky with age but that did not matter. I had never heard him sing before, although my mother had told me that once he was a wonderful singer. Such a voice was astonishing from such a frail old man. I listened, entranced, and saw how great he once was. His song opened a window through which I had a glimpse of his past and saw beyond the weak, elderly man to the person he used to be, notes still flowing. Although his voice sometimes faltered, the notes were rich and true, and his eyes were filled with a time and place that was unknown to me. I was mesmerized.

Other fragments of that day are all coming back to me now. I remember I was in a daze, a heightened state, as I had taken some pethidine that morning, for some reason. I was around sixteen years old. I often felt high. My mother often took me to our GP, ostensibly about a sore neck or period pains, but really about my high anxiety, and he happily wrote out another prescription for me. Perhaps he knew our family was a lost cause and could see the impact on me. Neither of them ever talked about this at these appointments; they just seemed to accept it was a normal thing to keep me in a state of chemical oblivion.

There was very little to inspire song in our house. This Sunday lunch was the extraordinary catalyst for the discovery of my own creativity. I remember writing my first-ever poem later that day, a significant moment for me. No ideas of using the arts as a means to express my feelings and life in this world were yet in my mind, but I was in a euphoric state. I was lifted out of myself. It was the first and only time I ever heard him sing. Below is that first poem.

The Singer

The spoiled chest heaves a sigh,
Summons remnants of a by-gone age
In the quavering, tentative notes
And in his eyes the beauty of the words,
And in his heart the singing of a bird.

The occasional fullness of velvet
Opens a window through which I look
With my mind breathing heavy,
And hear a young voice, doomed unknowing,
And see an old man, notes still flowing.

Listening to this memory singing to me, the importance of that brief moment of artistic expression and euphoria is clear. It is a beacon among the tall, separate trees of my family, showing me a place that I can go to when I am ready. And I do.

The more I write about how things were with me and share them with you, the more I realize what an enormous amount of emotion must have been stored in my gut. I have had many Upledger

CranioSacral Therapy sessions over twenty years and have progressed massively. Gradually, I am increasingly able to decipher the messages from my gut and understand them. Sometimes, though it is now rare, my gut is still unhappy, and sends me messages I need to listen to very carefully, and with a loving acceptance.

Loss of Kostek

I am sitting here wondering about writing some more neurological stuff, and I will, but another memory is looking hopefully at me. As I invite her to share with me, I can feel my gut tightening and an echo of nausea rising.

This memory is of myself as a young woman, divorced with two young children. I am in my little, terraced house that I grew to love dearly. This memory looks tired and hopeful as she shows me my mother who is now quite old. She has been diagnosed with Parkinson's disease and is very shaky, especially her hands and arms. She finds walking far to be very difficult and has stopped driving. By this time, I am practicing Upledger CranioSacral Therapy, and in spite of so many mixed emotions inside me, I offer her some treatment. She is now married to Pete, and he drives her over to see me. She lies down on my treatment couch, and I begin to work on her diaphragms—pelvic and respiratory, which are strong, transverse bands of fascia that create separation and stability in the body. These bands of fascia have a big impact on tension around the central nervous system and often hold emotional issues in their tissue. In our work, we facilitate, with a listening palpation, the release of patterns of tensions in these diaphragms. We gently give them an opportunity to unwind with our characteristically light touch.

My mother's shaking stops, and she relaxes. As I have my hands lightly on her respiratory diaphragm, she says she has something to tell me. She tells me this "something" in the way you might say, "Oh, apparently the price of carrots is going to double this week," as if there is nothing special to share. Then she tells me that Kostek, my biological father, has died, and she thought I might want to know. Nothing else is added to that statement. She closes her eyes again. Maybe she was in her own shame.

I am sitting in shock, in freeze, trying to process what I have just heard without showing my feelings and without feeling them. She says I "might have wanted to know" that my father had died? How could she have so massively underestimated the impact of this news on me?

I have been aware for a number of years that part of my drive to fulfill my potential used to come from a deep hope that Kostek might notice and consider me worthy of acknowledging in some small way. How I thought he would know what I was doing, I still have no idea, but I am aware of that as a past motivator. Sitting very still beside her, this news comes as a big shock because it signals the end of any possible opportunity or chance to ever meet him or hear from him.

The tears roll silently down my face and drop onto my lap. I cannot wipe my eyes as I still have both hands on my mother. This is such a metaphor for our relationship—me holding her and unable to attend to or express my own feelings. I carry on treating her, and she says nothing. I feel as if someone has burst a very big balloon of mine, and I am left with the broken pieces lying shriveled on my lap, not knowing what to do next.

After she has gone, I sink slowly into grief and despair. I feel a large ball of sorrow form inside me that has nowhere to express itself or be heard. Eventually it was heard, a few years later, during a multi-hands CranioSacral Therapy session. During that session, I put myself in my mother's shoes and imagined that I had this news to break to my own daughter. I visualized myself sitting beside my daughter, putting my arms around her, preparing to tell her the news with enormous sensitivity and compassion, reassuring her that I was there to listen to whatever she felt about this. I noticed how anxious I was about telling her and how I was dreading bearing a message that would cause her pain. Simultaneously, I saw that my mother had not experienced any of this and did not seem to have any idea of the impact her news might have on me. During that visualization, the tears fell freely from my eyes, and I witnessed the difference between my mother and myself. On the one hand, this difference is something to celebrate and, on the other, something to grieve over. But life is never simple, is it?

Not surprisingly, Kostek was never referred to again. This all happened a long time before the scuba diving accident. It was another "freeze" experience that built the tension in my gut and set the scene for the Post-Traumatic Stress Disorder that was to come as a result of the diving accident.

✳

Although my story involves early trauma and Post-Traumatic Stress Disorder with its associated gut problems, you do not need to have had either of these to benefit from reading these words. Life has many ways of throwing us challenges, from early family life, to events in our teenage and youth, and beyond. These challenges can be emotional, mental, spiritual, chemical, or physical, from disease, injury, or surgery. The more information we have, and the more we have some idea of how to start to listen to the inside world that is our body, the more likely we are to be able to change things in a positive way. If you are an Upledger CranioSacral therapist, your hands will become more informed, and perhaps you will be more aware of what might lie in the complex layers of the gastrointestinal tract and its enteric nervous system. If you are someone going to an Upledger CranioSacral therapist, more information will help your body show your hands where to work, and perhaps some of the exercises and ideas in this book will help you progress more swiftly toward better and more comfortable gut health. If you are someone who is drawn to this book just because you or someone near to you is suffering, I hope the information and practical side will be empowering, and, of course, I encourage you to find an Upledger CranioSacral therapist to help you on your journey.

6

SomatoEmotional
Release and Safety

The Universe is made of stories, not atoms.

MURIEL RUKEYSER

NEGATIVE FEELINGS AND THOUGHTS

Body tissues hold emotion, possibly from the beginning of our lives.

Our feelings are felt through our whole body. You can feel changes in levels of tension in your face and body when you are angry, sad, or happy. Some of these feelings—usually the negative ones—can remain in the body tissue. Negative emotions do not flow through us so readily as, say, love or joy. For instance, we may remember and hold on to negative experiences, so we do not repeat a certain behavior, such as eating a poisonous berry. This assures survival of the species. If someone is beaten, he or she will hold on to this memory to avoid it happening again. (Although, in reality, such avoidance is not always possible.)

Events in and around very young and not so young children can generate intense negative emotions, such as fear, anger, shame, loneliness, sadness, and guilt. These events do not need to happen directly or indirectly to young people to cause these feelings; they need only to happen in their surrounding environment. Young children may lack the awareness, safety, adult help, or verbal expertise to talk about these feelings.

With no way to release these feelings—either through verbal or physical expression—we protect ourselves by burying these feelings deep inside our bodies, somewhere they cannot cause so much pain. They create tension patterns and restrictions that, over the years, build up in layers and often lead to chronic pain, illness, or dysfunction. The event may pass, life may improve, but the emotion will stay buried in the body until something facilitates its release.

Our biography becomes our biology. Our whole emotional history is written throughout our body.

Thus holding on to negative experiences is not always helpful for our long-term health. Our mind sees everything through a hazy filter of these stored emotions that we may not even be aware of, and it sometimes reacts in strange and unhelpful ways—ways which may prevent us from having a healthy relationship with ourselves and with the other people in our lives. Our choices in life become very limited. Our joy and peace can be greatly diminished.

ENERGY CYSTS

Dr. John Upledger coined the term *energy cyst* to describe the process where the body can hold on to negative emotions felt as a result of a physical injury or emotional trauma, or both simultaneously. External energy, when forced into the body, is opposed only by the tissues' density, and it will penetrate as far as it can. It will then end up in a ball of disorganized energy, walled off from the tissue around it; this disorganized energy is what Dr. John called an *energy cyst*. Often, when the physical injury has healed, there are still problems if the energy cyst remains, as negative emotions may still be held there. This fits with the laws of thermodynamics that state that energy cannot be created or destroyed. These laws also tell us that the natural tendency of atoms, molecules, and energy is toward disorganization.

With the help of a skilled Upledger CranioSacral therapist, our bodies will often allow the energy to disperse. Any accompanying emotion and memories can then rise to the surface of our conscious awareness and release from our body, giving us back all the energy we have had to use to wall off that experience.

This energy is given back because CranioSacral Therapy, as with all effective and ethical therapy, works through facilitating self-awareness that is empowering and transforming. We, as Upledger CranioSacral therapists, never tell people what we think is going on, or what emotion we think might be buried where our hands are, or what might have caused their problems. That would be completely disempowering and very likely put the person on the table back several years in their therapeutic process. We remain grounded, blended with the person we are facilitating, and neutral—without judgment or agenda—in order to create a therapeutic space in which we listen and follow, and they feel safe enough to do the work they are ready to do in that session.

TECHNIQUES

Imagery and Visualization

When appropriate, Upledger CranioSacral therapists use the gentle and respectful approaches of SomatoEmotional Release in facilitating the release of emotions that may be held in the tissue. The imagery and visualization used in SomatoEmotional Release work can help create a clear image of what is happening in the body. Perhaps a pain or a very stuck place has a shape, a color, a texture, or a density that helps a person understand the emotion stored there and leads him or her to some kind of integration or resolution. The therapist creates a safe space that allows the person to explore and express these feelings, and the therapist's skilled hands allow the tissue's tension and dysfunction to release.

As well as gaining a better functioning and more relaxed central nervous system, these visualizations enable the person on the table to grow in awareness of the causes of what is happening to him or her and how to work with these causes going forward. He or she now has more choices and is therefore empowered in his or her life.

Two Inner Physicians

Upledger CranioSacral therapists are skilled facilitators, and the person on the table is the healer. The person's body-mind complex has all the skills, resources, and intelligence required to do this. Dr. John Upledger called this innate intelligence our "Inner Physician." But it can also be called our biological wisdom or higher self—the part of ourselves that carries our inner treatment plan. A session is facilitated by connecting the two Inner Physicians: that of the therapist/facilitator and that of the person on the table.

Upledger CranioSacral therapists believe that all parts of our body-mind system are conscious and have their story to tell. We often talk to the organs or parts of the brain of people who come to us, or even to groups of cells or parts of their system. There is much opportunity for our biological wisdom to speak through this work. Our clinical practice bears this out.

Significance Detector

We have a really helpful guide for what is significant for that person when he or she is talking to us. We call it the "Significance Detector." As we work with people, very often their craniosacral rhythm will suddenly stop. We sense they have dropped into a deeper and stiller place inside themselves—that their connection with their Inner Physician has become stronger and clearer.

The Significance Detector leads us to where that person's Inner Physician would like us to be at that moment. Perhaps the body is ready to show the person a memory, a feeling, or a place that needs attention. Dr. Upledger would encourage the person to explore this highly significant moment. We might ask, "What is in your awareness right now?" Or "How are you feeling at this moment?" This guide keeps us on track and grounded in the person's body-based process.

Dialoguing

Dialoguing can be done out loud with the person on the table to give voice to his or her Inner Physician or biological wisdom. Dialoguing can also occur silently by using the craniosacral rhythm and the Significance Detector to give the therapist yes-no answers. This is especially helpful for babies, very young children, or any nonverbal person. The information received is always invaluable and often quite unexpected. It comes from a place deeper than our rational, thinking mind. After all, if we could work out what was happening with the rational mind, we would all cure ourselves easily and without any help.

People are usually very open to connecting with this part of themselves and allowing that part to speak through them—especially if their journey toward better health has been long and difficult—as long as they feel safe with us. But it can be difficult or challenging at first for some people to set the rational mind to one side and access this part of their "non-conscious" (Dr. John's term for anything below our conscious awareness). This is where an experienced Upledger CranioSacral therapist can facilitate well. We are committed to ongoing work on ourselves in order to become more fully embodied and aware of our issues. We have opened up this pathway in ourselves over many sessions of SomatoEmotional release and are therefore better able to facilitate opening that pathway in the people who come to us. In this way, we can facilitate the growth in self-awareness that is essential to increased health and happiness.

These experiences and sensations inspired me to write a poem on fascia, that extraordinary fluid-filled connective tissue that communicates our history throughout our body and responds so readily to a grounded, neutral, and blended touch.

Fascia

Droplets strung like crystal beads along webs and
    ropes
Early morning dew, scattered bright necklaces on
    hedgerows
Fresh cool brooks and rivers outlining paths, fields,
    hill and valleys
Fluid landscape, quenching the earth's thirst
For stories, connections, information, growth

So in our bodies, the endless web of fascia
Living streams pouring through delicate networks
    of tissue
Whispering questions, answers,
Waters of the spirit, matrix of the soul
The most delicate tendrils reaching into every cell
surrounding every organ, muscle and bone,
Softly spoken provider of biological wisdom

Listen from a peaceful place
Gently travel the internal pathways

Rest awhile and breathe
Where the fascia is paused, unmoving,
Here perhaps a long-forgotten moment

Stay awhile and breathe.
Feel the body's story
Nourish the soul

SOMATOEMOTIONAL RELEASE SESSION

Here is what a SomatoEmotional Release session might look like. The person coming to the therapist lies on the treatment table or massage couch as usual. The therapist does a whole-body evaluation, listening to the craniosacral rhythm, checking for restrictions in the fascia, listening to tensions in the dural tube, and looking for energy cysts. The therapist will then be connected to the inner treatment plan of the person on the table and know where the person's Inner Physician would like them to start. The therapist will put his or her hands gently underneath and on top of the place the Inner Physician has revealed to them. He or she will then start blending, listening to, and following the tissue.

Sometimes the person on the table will begin to feel emotional. The therapist will explore this with open questions to facilitate their experience of this buried emotion, what it might be about and how the person can resolve any arising issues. Sometimes the person might feel a tension or block there. The therapist can facilitate his or her exploration of this by asking them if this block has a shape, color, texture, or density; how long it feels like it has been there;

what might have been going on at that time in his or her life that this block came to be there; what purpose it is serving for them; and similar questions. If the person on the table would like the block to go away, so the tissue can release after this exploration, which might include experiencing emotions as well, we facilitate the person's process to do this in any way that feels right for him or her.

Upledger CranioSacral therapists have no protocols or agendas save to meet that person where they are at that moment, without any intention to fix. In the end, it is always the person's choice of what to do with the session. The person on the table is the only person who can "fix" himself or herself, just as we, the therapists, can only work on ourselves and our own processes.

Indeed, without expressing and releasing the emotional component, any tissue release will be limited and probably temporary. I use SomatoEmotional Release every day in my clinic to facilitate releases in people who have carried old pain and emotion, sometimes for decades. It gives people choices and increases their self-awareness. It is CranioSacral Therapy at its richest, most powerful, and most empowering.

We trust this powerful and respectful SomatoEmotional process and follow it with compassion, empathy, and curiosity. The truth revealed to the person at that moment may not make sense to us, but it is his or her truth and experience, and as such, we validate it. This process will be resolved by the person by connecting to his or her biological wisdom—the Inner Physician. This often has physical, emotional, and spiritual facets.

These sessions may be very quiet and gentle; they may involve some tears, some talking, or some whole-body unwinding as the person on the table moves into positions helpful for releasing the tension patterns—perhaps reminiscent of the event they are exploring. Or they may happen in complete silence, as the person does his or her own emotional work with no need to talk to us during the process.

The person is always safe and in charge of the session and can decide what he or she wants to do at every moment. We, as therapists, always listen to the body and to the person and so will never explore what he or she does not want us to explore. We remain connected to his or her Inner Physician, who will show us the inner treatment plan that is right for that person on that day. Meeting the person exactly where he or she is, without an agenda, keeps the person safe and allows him or her to do what he or she needs to do in that session.

To be alongside another human being on a small part of his or her journey is an extraordinary experience for us as therapists. We feel deeply privileged to work in this way with our fellow human beings. To best do this work, it is imperative that we therapists have our own sessions and continue to work on our own processes in order to cleanly and safely facilitate other people's processes.

Neutral and Non-Knowing

As Upledger CranioSacral therapists, we remain, as I have said, grounded, blended with the person we are facilitating, and neutral, without judgment or agenda, in order to create a therapeutic space in which we listen and follow, and the person feels safe enough to do the work he or she is ready to do in that session. We aim to stay grounded in a state of "not knowing" rather than "knowing." After all, how can we really presume to know anything about the person on the table? Every human being is unique. If you line up ten people with migraines, for example, there will be ten different lists of causes and contributing factors. When we think we already know, we have no room in our awareness to learn. And our clients are not helped by such a mindset. As soon as we think we "know," we are lost.

Blending and Melding

The facilitating therapist and the person on the table often experience similar movements and changes in the body. Clearly, the emotional experience and its meaning are that of the person on the table, but when I rest my hands very gently on someone—grounding myself, breathing, neutral—the blending and melding with their tissues feels quite extraordinary. Sometimes suddenly, sometimes gradually, I am transported inside the world of his or her body—with all its different densities, textures, secret corners, movements, and stillness—with the sole task of listening to and following very carefully the stories there. It can feel as if my hands are inside the body, sensing areas of tension, pulls and twists, places that do not move and places that glide freely under my touch. The Inner Physician of the person seems to show me what I need to be aware of at that very moment. I might feel the bones, or the fascia, or the nerves, or the fluid flow come in turn into my hands, recruiting my help to unwind, release, unravel, and share the person's experience.

If there is a shift, a softening, a warmth growing, or a pulsing, it is not uncommon for the person and myself to comment on it simultaneously, as we experience the unfolding of the process. And it is through this listening and following that the tissues are given the opportunity to release any emotional component that is held there—whether by tears, laughter, or a memory of a person or an experience. Or sometimes the person on the table will do his or her emotional work in complete silence and privacy.

Sometimes it feels like a dance between me and the person on the table. I dance from my own body to his or hers. If I go too far into his or her body, I recognize this and come back more into my own. It is a constant, subtle shifting that demands of the therapist great awareness, focus, and grounding.

When it is my time to lie on the treatment table, I love experiencing this for myself. I feel the therapist's hands blend with me, and my body responds immediately, warming, unwinding, and releasing. Both of us go on a journey, driven and controlled by my Inner Physician, with no expectation of where we might end up—just a deep trust in the process of the incredible complexity that makes up every human being.

Through the process of CranioSacral Therapy and SomatoEmotional release, we can begin to change the oversensitivity in our nervous systems—central, autonomic, and enteric. We can begin to experience safety and to embed this in our cells.

SAFETY

Safety is the first fundamental requirement for someone to process his or her life experience as revealed by his or her body-mind complex. For many people with early childhood trauma, a feeling of being safe in the world is never really established, and so they are often in a heightened state of fight or flight, or, worse still, freeze. When things become completely overwhelming, they are triggered into these states very quickly. If their default in their central nervous system is fight or flight, their amygdala overreacts often and quickly, as their sympathetic nervous system kicks in swiftly and/or their reticular activating system is constantly triggered. If they are sometimes in freeze, they shut down and often dissociate, as their parasympathetic system—specifically the dorsal vagal complex—goes into overdrive.

Many people of all ages live their lives in a state of tissue tension and anxiety; they are often hypervigilant, as their body is in a protective state, a state of survival. Perhaps their pericardium has tightened around their heart to prevent further heartbreak.

Perhaps their gut has become inflamed, dysfunctional, oversensitive, and tense.

When I experience fear, I feel a wave of fear wash through my whole bowel and small intestine, all the way up to my respiratory diaphragm. I felt fear as I sat down to talk to you today, fear that I would run out of words, fear that my words would be meaningless, fear that this book will not resonate with anyone but me! This fear is born of that old isolation and the experience of not being okay or good enough or able to manage being in this world. Hello, my old friend. As the fear rolls through the tissue, I become tense and full of self-doubt and anxiety. I often wonder if I am alone in this, so I want you to know that if you have ever experienced this or something like it, you are not alone.

When I feel this happening, I question what it is that I am afraid of and talk to my gut; I put my hands on it and attempt to put the fear into perspective. It is usually out of proportion with the actual thought or event triggering its arrival. I recognize that the fear I feel is resonating back through the years to my scuba diving accident and to all my early life experience. It is as if once it is felt, it gathers up into a great big bundle of terror, of all the fear I have ever felt. All the cells in my gut carrying a memory of the old fear begin to shake and jump up and down, as if I am about to die. Increasingly now, I talk to them gently, silently, to reassure them that I am no longer in a dangerous situation and that they can relax and feel safe. These cells like being talked to like this. They respond well and often my gut calms down, and I become more grounded and relaxed.

Through the process of CranioSacral Therapy and SomatoEmotional release, we can begin to change the oversensitivity in our nervous systems—central, autonomic, and enteric. We can begin to have the experience of safety and to embed this in our cells.

SHUTDOWN

This brings us to another aspect of safety. Many people who come to us, having felt safe in their lives, often find this work doubly difficult. Their paradox is this: they are very shut down—their emotions are deeply buried in their tissues, and they have a strong, rational mind keen to control the situation—and yet they are most in need of opening that pathway to the deeper part of themselves. They will often display a strong resistance to their therapist's facilitating this. This is quite normal, and I find it frequently in my clinic. My ability to create a safe and nonjudgmental space for them is our starting point. Until they feel safe enough at a deep level, nothing will happen. The most helpful things I can offer to someone to create safety are my work on myself, my ability to be grounded (fully in my body), my palpation skills, my blending with his or her body-mind complex, and my neutrality. Once this is established, the work can begin.

FEAR

The tissues express strain and tension patterns that inhibit good fluid flow and healthy functioning of all aspects of the craniosacral system. To create safety for ourselves and for the people who come to us, it is helpful to understand more deeply how our body responds to danger at a cellular level and which mechanisms remember these experiences.

Where do you feel fear most in your body? How does your gut respond when you are afraid? It seems a great deal of fear is held in the gut's cell memory. It seems the cells are remembering fear and reacting with fear as a first response.

Dr. John always knew our cells held memories. His knowing did not always come from theories or books but from his clinical and personal experience working with himself and others. There is more and more research coming out to show this is the case.

> *If you want others to be happy, practice compassion. If you want to be happy, practice compassion.*
>
> DALAI LAMA

Case Story—Peter
Establishing Safety and Letting the Patient Lead the Way

Peter was a ten-year-old boy brought to me by his mother. He had an unusual history of speech development issues from the age of two years old and severe constipation from the age of six years old. At the time I first met Peter, he was on four sachets of Movicol (a laxative) per day just to keep his bowels moving regularly. He had constant headaches and dizziness. His speech was limited in expressive ability. In spite of all this, he was a very active boy who loved football and had a very friendly, positive outlook on life. His mother was very caring and nurturing and, not surprisingly, very worried about him.

Upon hands-on evaluation, the first thing I noticed was how difficult it was for him to be still and to be touched for any length of time. I would begin around the bottom of his spine, his sacrum, and the pelvic diaphragm, and work my way up to his neck. He would move and wriggle his body away from me. He was very willing to be treated, but it was as if his body could not bear what was happening.

The closer to his neck, the more uncomfortable it was for him. When I approached his neck and cranial base, it was almost impossible for him to let me work there, even if I was barely touching him. His occiput (the bone at the back and base of the skull) and his neck were very sensitive and extremely tense. It seemed he was in pain if I made any gentle attempt to listen with my hands, even with a blended and neutral touch, to what was happening there. Most of my work that was acceptable to him was on the gut, listening carefully to the layers and facilitating whatever release I could.

As we worked together over the next few months, there were slight improvements. Peter came off the Movicol and his bowels, although far from perfect, were at least working on their own. I also encouraged his mother to give him probiotics. His headaches diminished, and his dizziness was absent most of the time. His neck was still incredibly tight and sensitive, however.

Peter saw a pediatrician to evaluate his neck. An MRI was done as well as X-rays. Some abnormalities were found.

I began working in his mouth as well. Peter found this extremely difficult, and we would negotiate how long I would stay in one place before coming out. He would agree to let me work in his mouth for a count of three or five. I would count slowly and calmly out loud, so he knew when it would come to an end. He seemed to be in pain when I worked inside his lower teeth, at the sides in the soft tissue, and at the base of his tongue. As I worked with my little finger gently on the roof of his mouth, sending my intention through the hard palate to the vomer, to the sphenoid, and to the pituitary nestling in the middle of the sphenoid in the Sella Turcica, or turkish saddle, he was able to breath more easily and to cope with my presence there. This mouth work gradually became a little easier for him and his symptoms alleviated further.

I also taught him how to breathe more deeply. I asked him to do tongue stretching exercises as he was not able to lick his lips when I first met him, as his tongue was so tense. I also asked him to chew his food at least twelve times each mouthful, as he would just swallow whatever was in his mouth very quickly.

It became apparent that Peter had a sensory processing dysfunction. He was anxious and often in fight or flight. His tactile sensitivity, anxiety, visual sensitivity (he would not maintain eye contact for very long and told me it hurt his eyes to do so), oral sensitivity, and possibly auditory issues all pointed to this. On my recommendation, his mother ordered him a heavy weighted blanket that was calming and integrating for the central nervous system. His love of exercise, mostly football, would fit with this picture as any heavy work for the muscles has a calming and integrating effect on the whole sensory processing system. And when you consider that 80 percent of what our brain does is sensory processing, this is extremely important.

The CranioSacral Therapy, mostly working on his vagus nerve and his gut-brain connection, gradually allowed Peter to have a well-functioning gut and better ability to relax.

This Story's Message

Peter's story illustrates the impact of a very tight neck and occipital cranial base, which compromised the good function of the vagus nerve, impacting his ability to rest and to digest his food easily.

7

The Black Hole

This morning, my throat is pulling down into my respiratory dia-phragm, and my gut is still and heavy. I see a memory that has been trying to get my attention. She has very dark circles under her eyes. Her eyes are circles of pain. Empty orbs of blue, empty of tears, empty of love, they see nothing at all but thick black despair. I can hardly bear to look at her, to look at myself at that age. She reminds me of our darkness. This is the darkest black you can imagine, no chink of light anywhere, endless and infinite. No stars in this firmament, no sun to rise or moon to wish upon. This blackness presses up against every part of my skin, seeps through the skin and invades and fills every cell in my body, and darkens every corner of my mind. It suffocates me. There is no room for anyone else in this black. And who would want to be here? I am shocked to find myself here. I am terrified of my only option. Is this memory of the first time in my life my choices were reduced to just one? I think back to the baby that refused to eat; that was the first time. The only way out was to die, to let go of life. With that on my mind, I found my pethidine and phenobarbitone.

It was a Saturday morning, and I was at home. I remember my mother was not in the house. I was sixteen years old and in my first sixth form year at school. I was the youngest in my year. Alfred must have been out somewhere too. No one to disturb me, I fetched a glass of water and took the tablets carefully, one at a time, not in a rush, but mindfully touching, holding, and swallowing each one. I waited to slip away.

There was no fear any more, just a relief at a decision made, waiting for oblivion in the silence. There was a long, slow pause. I sat down. Minutes passed. I didn't know how many and time didn't seem to matter anymore. Somewhere a long way away in the distance, I heard a phone ring. It was insistent. It penetrated my black world. Something in me needed to answer it. Strange.

I picked up the phone and soon felt my blurred mind inhibiting my speech. It was Jenny, my best friend, who did not live far away. I have no idea what words were exchanged. She worked out what I had done. An unfathomable time after that, Jenny and her mother came to my house and found me, sleepy and confused. They bundled me up, put me in their car, and rushed me to the hospital. My stomach was pumped. I was left to sleep. My boyfriend came to see me with a friend of his sometime afterward and unceremoniously dumped me for what I had done. He watched me for sadness or complaint. I had none of these for him. I had no energy for emotion any longer. There was even a slight bemusement that he could think this was all about him. He was of the smallest significance.

My mother came to pick me up later and told me crossly that it was inconvenient to come and pick me up, and that it was a very silly thing I had done. That was the end of any conversation with her.

I saw a psychiatrist the week after, and he asked me why I took the pills. I said because I wanted to go to sleep. He took me literally and asked me why I did not ask my doctor for sleeping pills and signed me off. He did not hear that I wanted to go to sleep forever and never wake up. That was the end of that conversation and all conversations.

The only support I remember was from my classics teacher the next week at school. She saw how pale and thin I was and asked me if I was alright. I found myself telling her what had happened that weekend. She was compassionate and said how brave I was to come into school that week. It was a wonderful thing to hear and probably one of the few times I had a positive comment at that time in my life. I still feel so grateful for her words.

From that day, my nervous systems—central, autonomic, and enteric—was overwhelmed. They were being asked to hold on to so many unexpressed feelings that they were not able to function well. My anxiety levels rose higher than ever. My hands shook all the time. I could no longer pick up a glass full of water without spilling it. I did not even try to pick up hot drinks. I could only drink these when I was by myself. I would hold the cup with both hands, leave the cup barely on the table, and bend my head down to reach the cup. In this awkward position, I would take one small sip at a time. I felt ashamed. If I was in the company of anyone else, when I had a cold drink I would need to use two hands. It was still a shaky and uncertain procedure that filled my stomach with butterflies every time I attempted to take a drink. This lasted for years, this shakiness. I cannot remember when it stopped. Probably very gradually over the next fifteen years or so.

Am I glad I did not succeed? Yes, wholeheartedly.

This morning I was driving to the hairdresser and was overwhelmed by the sky. Pinks and oranges glowed almost unbearably brightly through streaks of stretched out white and gray clouds, threaded tapestry like across the early blue sky. All of this offers my soul a reason to be here. There's more. This skyscape rises triumphantly over a cold mist, laid over the grass fields like dark, moist cotton wool. It's a mist that brings the black silhouetted trees to stillness and silence. I am in awe. I am filled with joy.

If I had succeeded all those years ago, I would have missed this and so many beautiful experiences—and above everything else, my two children.

Memories: Overwhelm and Shame

I notice there are a group of red-faced memories looking at me and turning away every time I meet their gaze. They are embarrassed and ashamed. Ah yes, of course, I see what they are telling me. At this time in my life, I blush and turn bright burning red in the face whenever I am a little embarrassed or put on the spot. The redness lasts for hours. Everyone can see it and there is nothing I can do to make it go away more quickly. Of course, no one says anything—nor do I. My life is mostly lived behind a brick wall of protection and isolation.

My mind is now filled with sounds of my childhood and teen-age years. Tears, both mine and my mother's, filled my life. Alfred's tears were always silent. My mother often sobbed violently on her bed. I cried in my room more quietly, for longer and more often. My mother and Alfred shouted at each other from across the din-ing table during meals and other times throughout the house. They would throw accusations at each other, yelling and calling each other names that were abusive and insulting. I hear the music I played— all of Leonard Cohen's melancholy songs, cello concertos, requiem masses, the Moody Blues, Beatles, and Rolling Stones—these were all great escapes and soothed me often.

Very often, when it was unbearable to be at home, I would leave the house and walk along the busy roads at night. I walked for miles, going nowhere. No one asked where I was going or when I would be back. Even a superficial show of care might have built a bridge into a deeper conversation. My mother did everything in her power to avoid that. And, in reality, she was only ever concerned about herself.

The memory who is telling me this story has wet, straggly long hair, and her mascara is running down her face. She takes my hand and places it carefully on her face. I feel her icy, wet young skin. I gently stroke her forehead and push her fringe back out of her eyes. I feel very sad. I gently put my hand on her abdomen and feel it is as tight as a board. She looks thin, cold, and soaking wet, and she reminds me that these walks were frequently in the rain. I remember the feel of the rain on my face. It mingled with the tears that ran down my cheeks, washed them away and cooled my hot, puffy eyes. Through my tears and the rain on the wet road, the lights of the cars are scattered and streaked. The lights are white and red, and they make it hard to focus. I do not want to focus. I am still looking for oblivion, looking for a way to avoid my pain, to find some comfort, some relief. My long night walks were so full of sensory experiences—the rain, the light, the sound of the cars louder and softer as they passed me—that distracted my brain for a while. I loved the feeling they gave me.

Eventually, even after witnessing the pain Pete caused me, my mother married him, and many of the sounds did not change. I only lived with them for one year in his house. My mother sold the house I lived in with her and Alfred. The other difference was the regular sound of wood pigeons. Even now, when I hear these birds I am dragged unwillingly back to that house, to that time. It is an almost unbearable feeling of dread that fills my entire gut.

One big difference between Peter and Alfred was that Pete was louder, less intelligent, and more abusive than Alfred. He was also frequently violent. I'd guess that he was with his first wife, and was probably either violent or sexually abusive to his daughters as well. He would often hit my mother repeatedly, knocking her to the floor. This violence continued until he was too old to be bothered with the physicality of the beatings, and then he just shouted, yelled, and threw things. Every single time this happened my mother would turn to me for sympathy, understanding, and help. I was so angry every time that she did this. She married Pete knowing he was violent and also knowing how much he had hurt me. She was a harsh, disapproving, and demanding woman, who endlessly provoked Alfred and then Pete. She was unkind and neglectful to me my whole life. Even after I moved out, she would call me to complain and tell me every detail about the latest violent incident—expecting me to be sorry for her. She would sob on the phone and say she had no one else to talk to. She wanted me to blame Pete for everything and give her sympathy. I had none and could not wait to hang up.

This pattern of asking me for sympathy was familiar. When my mother and Alfred argued, they would come individually into my room and do their best to persuade me to take their side as they gave me a heated description of all the personality flaws of the other one. They somehow wanted me to say they were right, they were the good person; the other one was bad and had done wrong. When one of them left my room, the other would come in a little later and do the same thing. They would both berate me for not being sympathetic and not taking sides. I never took sides. How could I, when each was as bad as the other? I just listened to them both, feeling my insides tie themselves into a tight knot. Neither of them was ever concerned about the impact their constant battles might have on me. Neither of them ever considered that they might play a part in this war and that perhaps they needed to learn how to communicate better. I did not make these suggestions for two reasons: first, because I would be shouted at for being so rude, and second, because I had no idea what the problems were. I knew nothing about communicating feelings, only how to store them in my body. In that I was becoming an expert.

Relationships

By this point in my life, I had never witnessed any adult communication or seen two adults in a healthy relationship, except perhaps a glimpse at a friend's house, where I watched her parents hug each other. I watched them in amazement and embarrassment—it was such an unusual sight. So often, I fell at the first hurdle in all my relationships with men and women. I was unable to make a secure or close attachment to a female friend or a boyfriend due to my early history, which had left me with a very underdeveloped ventral vagal complex. This complex often left me in fight, flight, or freeze. As soon as I began to feel close to someone, huge fear and insecurity would rise up, often unrecognized by me for what it was, and I was unable to relax or engage with that person; I felt incredibly awkward, shy, self-conscious, and alienated. Not surprisingly, my relationships did not last very long. Other girls my age seemed confident, happy, and relaxed. They were like aliens to me. I was the opposite—insecure, often sad, always tense, and anxious. Having never witnessed two people in a harmonious relationship in my family, there was a big chasm to jump across to find that harmony, connection, and ease of communication. I had no idea how to make that jump and make friends, of which I only ever had very few.

As I look back, I am grateful that there were a few people who befriended me in spite of my ineptitude. I remember some incidents in which my shame and inability to talk honestly or openly left me in a silent, frozen place where no one could reach me. I can still feel the embarrassment remembering these situations. I saw everyone's attitude toward me through heavy filters of expected deceit and rejection. My first boyfriends must have found me very insecure and anxious and often silent when there were feelings to be expressed but no words to enable this expression. Male friendships were always the most difficult. I often felt delighted if they wanted to spend time with me but then was equally terrified that I would be so boring or disappointing that they would regret it.

This has changed immeasurably over my journey with Upledger CranioSacral Therapy, and I want you, reader, to know that however difficult life has been, we are all capable of change and increased health and happiness. Always stay open to the possibility of your life becoming better and your gut more comfortable. I see human beings as the unfolding of infinite possibilities. And now, I have an image of the beautiful lotus flower unfolding in my mind's eye.

You may be wondering how Upledger CranioSacral Therapy helped me forge relationships. It was through finding a safe space with the many truly wonderful, compassionate therapists who stayed with me for as long as it took to reach the buried feelings and find a way to express them. This enabled me to gain a better understanding of my past and insight into how it created my present existence. I began slowly making friends with colleagues in the Upledger world who had a level of wisdom and kindness that was so encouraging and heartfelt; they made my first faltering steps into connection possible. I am eternally grateful to all of them. My colleagues and friends in this world are my family, my tribe.

I was able to see that it was the adults in my life who were flawed, and I was simply an innocent child in a very difficult situation. Gradually, I began the long journey of building self-esteem. Gradually, I took down the wall that protected me, one brick at a time.

My relationship with my children evolved into one that is open, loving, close, and supportive. It has become an enormous part of my healing process. Interestingly—although not so surprisingly perhaps, given our knowledge of how connected parents and their children are physiologically—it was the work I did on myself that shifted things between myself and my two children. I have seen this happen in families many times over the years. When parents do their inner work, their children change automatically. The dynamic in the relationships between the family members shifts into one that is more positive and healthy. It is never enough to work only with the baby or child. This is limiting and superficial compared with the riches gained when the whole family is open to doing their work and to change. Life is magical.

8

Still Frozen?

Cells and Our Family Trees

Frozen Potential

In the shower this morning, as I lift my face and feel the water spraying warm and cleansing across my skin, the panic begins to rise in my stomach. Panic always comes. My fight or flight is triggered. Everything below my respiratory diaphragm tightens and lifts. I gasp and move my face out of the water as my body moves quickly into freeze. My heart thumps, and I spend a few minutes focusing on calming my breathing. Flashbacks are never far from the surface—hanging in the deep, cold sea, unable to breathe, water in my throat. This is how my day starts. This is a morning ritual.

I think of other things—what I am going to have for breakfast, what I am going to wear. Still, my body is afraid. I tell my body I am not in danger; I am in the shower; it is okay. I am so weary of having this conversation every morning. My cells keep holding on to the memory, just in case.

I have been ready for danger most of my life. I see danger everywhere. I am also very courageous and do not let this stop me from moving forward, being adventurous, but it is an uncomfortable paradox.

Writing this book, I realize how often I still go into freeze in my autonomic nervous system. I catch myself more often now with a still tension in my body, a quiet ache in the gut, my breath shallow and silent. Even now, apparently, my body-mind sometimes wants to be invisible and inaudible. For years, I was unaware of how often this would happen. Looking outside after my shower, I see a very cold, frozen world, mirroring my internal state.

Leaving all chores behind me, I head out into this icy place toward the river. The cold air freshens me as I inhale, and I enjoy the white cloud I puff out of my mouth with each exhale. The skin on my face quickly cools, and there is a clarity that comes with the cold. Meeting the river, my breath is taken away momentarily by the beauty in front of me. The water shines thickly like a rippled mirror, slightly misted by the breath of a cold winter night. Strange, slender twists of cold rise from its surface, as if they are hugging their arms around themselves in the frost, and this makes them separate from the rest. The color palette is full of whites, blues, grays, and deep greens, shifting and blending inside an oil painting still being created by an unseen artist of extraordinary talent. All potential is held here, unmoving, hiding, waiting for something to happen. Perhaps this is what it is like when you or I go into freeze. All potential is held, unmoving, hiding, waiting for something to happen, waiting for enough safety to unlock all of this. I catch my breath again, absorbing every detail of this frozen scene to memory. There is beauty even in freeze.

LIMBIC SYSTEM ON SPEED DIAL

Memory feels so complex and somehow almost out of my control. That is because experiences that are intense and overwhelming are sometimes not processed and filed neatly away in our hippocampus, along with other experiences. They become stuck in the amygdala. As with any post-traumatic stress, the amygdala in our brain's limbic system (the part of the brain associated with emotional experience and family) is easily triggered, and the body reacts instantly. It becomes, as I heard somewhere, the Patron Saint of Overreaction. This makes me smile. We do not know how to process these overwhelming experiences, and they remain powerful, unsettling; they often create flashbacks and intrusive memories. Our amygdala becomes larger and our hippocampus smaller. The pathways firing during these reactions become well-trodden—like a path through a forest that has been walked many times over the years. Because of this, our responses fly through our body-mind in a flash.

To forge a new path takes time. We have to decide to take a different path every time we walk through the forest, and we must do so for a long time. It takes a lot of energy to create a new path, and making this choice over and over again can be tiring. But is anyone else equally exhausted from finding themselves running down the route with the flattened grass and firm soil, too overcome to go back to find the new route?

Sitting here, talking to you, my heart is thumping, reminding me to be careful, telling me there might be danger around the corner, preparing me for an unseen disaster.

I am wondering what happens in our second brain each time the responses of the body-mind are triggered in this way. How does our enteric nervous system react? We know it communicates with the vagus nerve, which is a big part of our autonomic nervous system, and so when the enteric nervous system receives this message of danger it will either go into high alert or freeze. We also know the enteric nervous system sends messages about the state of our gut—including the long tube and the state of the microbiota—back to the brain via our vagus nerve. The enteric nervous system also communicates with the sympathetic branch of the autonomic nervous system via the prevertebral ganglia. In fact, there are many more messages going from gut to brain than the other way around. But the enteric nervous system will not share all of its experience with our central nervous system and autonomic nervous system. As a complicated system that can process massive amounts of data, it also has complete reflex circuits that enable it to make its own decisions. This is why it is often referred to as the second brain. Surely, then, the enteric nervous system can be thought of as part of the peripheral nervous system only by definition; in terms of anatomy and function, it can be considered another branch of the autonomic nervous system.

Traditionally, anatomists and physiologists have taught us there are two branches to the autonomic nervous system, the sympathetic and the parasympathetic. The sympathetic is our fight or flight system that prepares us to face danger, so we can run away or fight whatever is threatening us. This system takes blood away from our digestive system and sends it to our muscles; it opens our airways, so we can breathe harder if we need to run away from danger. This system uses a lot of energy and speeds our metabolism. The parasympathetic is our rest and digest system. It allows us to digest our food, store our energy, and switch off and rest calmly. The vagus nerve, cranial nerve X, is a big part of our parasympathetic system. When we consider that the autonomic nervous system actually has three branches—the sympathetic, the parasympathetic, and the enteric nervous system—it is clear that the situation is more complex than previously understood. If we include polyvagal theory, with its two branches of the vagus nerve, the autonomic nervous system can be thought of as having four branches.

We are sitting at a crossroads, you and I, as our discussion can go in two different directions. We can look more closely at the autonomic nervous system and its new complexity to see what light this sheds on how our body responds to our life. Or we can examine cells and cell memory.

It feels as if I am sitting in front of a large canvas with brushes of all sizes and every color beside me. Shall I pick up the broad brush or the slender, tiny ones?

I am going to pick up the broad brush and paint with bold, sweeping strokes in an attempt to paint the big picture, to integrate some of this into a whole that we can begin to understand and work with. Then, we can enhance our painting with microscopic details regarding the cells in our guts and how they sense and remember our experiences.

AUTONOMIC NERVOUS SYSTEM

Think again of the long tube that is our digestive tract—beginning with our mouth, then becoming our esophagus, stomach, duodenum, small intestine, bowel, and anus—nearly nine meters in length. The gastrointestinal tract is the largest external surface of our body. Everything inside it is actually part of the outside world, and it is only when we absorb some of the contents through its wall and into ourselves that the contents of the digestive system are inside our body. Take a moment to let that sink in.

We bring the outside world into ourselves through the gastrointestinal tract, the long tube. How do we respond to the world? Do we embrace or resist it? Do we receive it peacefully or in a state of tension? The gastrointestinal barrier is the moment of decision to allow in or to not allow in. It is where we hover between two worlds: our inner world and the outside world. It represents so much more than the absorption of nutrients from food. It is part of our emotional, physiological, and mental response to our outside world. Our reaction here, in between the two worlds, affects everything, from tiny individual cells to our enteric nervous system, our autonomic nervous system, our central nervous system, and our immune and endocrine systems, which are inextricably linked to the enteric nervous system in our gut.

How we respond to the world in which we find ourselves is affected by the generations preceding us—our mother, father, their parents, and their parents—as well as the nature of our existence. In fact, there are so many threads woven into the beautiful, rich fabric of existence that it is beyond my comprehension. I don't have all the answers, and I don't think anyone does yet, so I can only offer my wonder and curiosity as I take your hand to explore some of this in the hope that you will be inspired to ask questions without the need for clear answers. The intricacy is a delight to be marveled at rather than fretted over. It can lead us to become less limited in our thinking about our lives and our health and, as a result, to be more open to the possibility of understanding and healing. So let's not fret, you or me, about trying to pin it all down neatly. Let's enjoy the journey.

While I still have my broad paintbrush in my hand, let's look in a little more detail at Stephen Porges's polyvagal theory, as his theory and new ideas about the vagus nerve add richness to our understanding of the autonomic nervous system and show that this system may be more adaptable, or "plastic," than we have realized up to this point. Porges developed this theory after many years of researching the vagus nerve, and the theory is expanding our view of our autonomic nervous system in many ways, including helping us to realize that ideally humans can transition between the different states of their nervous system as required by their current situation.

We looked at how Porges describes the vagus nerve having two branches, not just one. The different branches I am discussing here are clearly illustrated in the diagram of the new model of the autonomic nervous system (p. 63). One is the dorsal vagal complex, the oldest branch of the vagus nerve. The dorsal nucleus of the vagus nerve lies on the floor of the fourth ventricle in the medulla oblongata. The four ventricles are the spaces inside our brain that contain most of our cerebrospinal fluid and are also where the cerebrospinal fluid is produced. The dorsal vagal complex innervates and controls primarily the viscera below the respiratory diaphragm, including the gastrointestinal tract. The dorsal vagal tract is not myelinated, so messages are slower, and it is concerned with primal survival. It is found in most animals. When under great stress and threat, the dorsal vagal complex is the part of the vagus nerve that takes us into freeze—playing dead, conserving energy, and slowing the metabolism. Under normal conditions, the dorsal vagal complex regulates the digestive processes. However, if it is not balanced by any other part of the vagal system over a period of time, it can result in potentially lethal conditions, such as apnea (cessation of breathing) and bradycardia (very slow heart rate). It is all about balance!

The other branch of the vagus system is the ventral vagal complex. This is the vagal tract that Porges believes to be a more recent development, evolutionarily speaking. Mammals, such as humans, are becoming increasingly complex neurologically over time; we have evolved a more sophisticated system to adapt to and create behavioral and emotional responses to our increasingly complex world. The ventral nucleus originates in the nucleus ambiguous in the medulla oblongata. The medulla oblongata is a continuation of the spinal cord at the bottom of the brain and is found in front of the cerebellum. Its actions are involuntary, and we cannot live without it. It controls breathing, swallowing, and heart rate, as well as myriad other important functions. The ventral vagal complex is myelinated for fast and speedy adaptation and response. It talks to the viscera above the respiratory diaphragm, including the soft palate, pharynx (so influencing speech and swallowing), larynx, esophagus, and bronchi. It is concerned with social engagement and social attachment behaviors. It puts the brakes on our fight or flight response, not letting our heart rate speed up into fight or flight mode. It allows us to self-soothe and calm.

Interestingly, the nucleus of the facial nerve, cranial nerve VII, lies on the edge of the nucleus ambiguous, and the sensory aspects of the trigeminal nerve (which innervates the temporomandibular joint that allows us to open and close our mouth) come into the nucleus ambiguous. Both these nerves are involved in the ventral vagal complex and therefore in the expression and experience of a range of emotion.

Our talk about paths through forests applies here. We all have our established default setting, or well-trodden path, in terms of the autonomic nervous system. How is this created? It is created through our interactions as a baby, both in utero and after birth, with our environment, with our mother, and with other adults involved in our care that develop the ventral vagal complex to a greater or a lesser extent. The National Institutes of Health published a paper on infant child development in February 2011, titled "The Early Development of the Autonomic Nervous System Provides a Neural Platform for Social Behavior; A Polyvagal Perspective."[18] Recall that multigenerational influences also play a part here.

Consider again a baby who has a mother who lacks emotional intelligence, resilience, the ability to articulate her emotions, or the ability to make safe attachments to adults as a child, or friends and partners as an adult. This mother is often in fight and flight and feels unsafe, possibly in freeze some of the time. How will that baby's ventral vagal complex be developed? Its mother will not have a well-tuned ventral vagal complex. If the mother or prime carer does not have a well-developed and functioning ventral vagal complex, she will not engage with her child in a way that will develop theirs. The baby will become a child and then an adult lacking in affiliative social skills, therefore lacking the ability to regulate their fight or flight responses.

Knowing how plastic our nervous system is, there is always hope to change this over time with the right input—perhaps an intervening adult who has those skills, a compassionate teacher at school, a helpful counselor, or of course, an Upledger CranioSacral therapist incorporating SomatoEmotional Release. In this way, we can always mitigate the effects of generational influences on ourselves and so change things for our children and their children.

It comes back to the fundamental concept of safety that we talked about earlier. Our nervous system is constantly responding to environmental cues and judging how safe we are. If we feel safe, our ventral vagal complex and/or dorsal vagal complex will be engaged; if we feel threatened, our sympathetic fight or flight response will be engaged, and the ventral vagal complex and dorsal vagal complex will be inhibited. Remember that the sympathetic system is in regular communication with the enteric nervous system. If we feel so unsafe that we think we might die, what happens to the gut? Our dorsal vagal complex takes us into freeze. Remember, the dorsal vagal complex is primarily connected with the gut, so consider the consequences when we are in freeze. If we are in freeze, we need time and space to feel safe enough to come out of freeze—probably into fight or flight; someone can then approach us through the ventral vagal complex. You cannot talk someone into feeling safe if they are in freeze; just being with them quietly is more helpful. They need space and time. If someone is in fight or flight, however, you might be able to socially engage with them and calm them down through your ventral vagal complex.

Polyvagal theory gives us many insights into working with people with trauma. Being in the ventral vagal complex is a goal for many but not necessarily everyone, especially perhaps for people on the autism spectrum who may prefer to stay predominantly in the dorsal vagal complex. We have much to learn.

It appears to be all about degrees of safety. Whether it's our anatomy, cell memory, or my personal story, everything comes back to feeling safe, to survival, which is closely connected with our enteric nervous system. The fibers of the dorsal vagal complex connect into the enteric nervous system, as does the sympathetic nervous system. If our central nervous system is neuroplastic and glial plastic, surely our enteric nervous system must also be neuroplastic and glial plastic. There are possibilities, then, to work with the gut's own nervous system in a way similar to how people who have been injured by stroke or accident or trauma can work with the plasticity of their brain to regain function. This gives us hope for ourselves, for anyone reading this who feels hopeless, and for the people that come to us as Upledger CranioSacral therapists.

Memory: Tightly Wound Nineteen-Year-Old

I am sitting here wondering how I will add those details to the picture I am painting for you. My intention last night was to next discuss cells and their responses and capacity for memory, but that is not what is calling me today. You remember my shadows? My memories? A few have come forward and shared their stories. Well, there is one now, a little separate from the group. She has furrows in her brow and her shoulders are tense and hunched. She is pacing up and down somewhere in my mind. I am trying to see her face more clearly to see how old she is. It is difficult to tell, as she is constantly moving. I think she is around nineteen years old. As she goes to and fro, I become aware of the front of her body. It looks like a metal spring or spiral fills her abdominal space; it has been wound up and cannot unwind, as it is trapped inside her. It reminds me of a silver metal slinky.

The spring looks like a child's drawing, where they have taken a pencil and drawn the spiral impatiently, going faster and faster until the center is a mess of lines and smudges. There is also a feeling of never-ending movement. Somehow the drawing is never finished; never at peace; constantly being worked on and worked over, over and over again. Some of the other memories approach her, but she seems cold and does not respond. This is not because she is cold or detached. She is bound up with anxiety, and every time she makes an attempt at reaching outside herself, this pulls her back inside to her private turmoil.

Her gut is in a constant state of tension, expressed sometimes in cramps, sometimes in nausea, sometimes in butterflies in her stomach. It feels as if this metal spiral has been threaded through all the parts of her bowel, small intestine, stomach, and esophagus, reacting to every tightening by the unseen hand of some kind of surgeon. Sometimes she can't breathe properly, and her heart starts thumping. Sometimes she wants to weep. Sometimes she despairs. Have you ever felt like this? I hope and believe I am not the only one.

At nineteen years old, I could never share what I was feeling. There was no one I felt comfortable and safe enough with to make myself so vulnerable. The thought that you are reading this now is strange, but I think now is the time to be honest. How can I talk to that memory as she paces up and down? How can I tell her to just stop for a moment to let me see her? To really see her? I can let her know it is okay to feel how she feels and that how she feels does not make her any less valuable than anyone else on this planet. I can encourage her to talk to me, to let me put my arms around her for a moment. Holding her—feeling her anxious body, her bony skeleton tightly bound with muscle and ligament—may be painful, but it has to be better than leaving her pacing in my head the rest of my life.

I know why she appeared today. Last night, she was active all night in my body-mind. I was restless, and my mind would not stop overthinking and stressing over everything in my life. My body ached. I was hot, and then I was cold. I was over the duvet, then under the duvet. My whole self is filled with the tension of this metal spiral. Still, after so many years, it can impact me and stir my tissue memory.

How ironic! She has led us to where we began! Time to look at our cells, especially the cells in the gut. How do they respond to our experience? Can they really remember it? As an Upledger CranioSacral therapist I know the concept of tissue memory to be true. It is at the center of all our work to trust in the biological wisdom of the body; to know that the body remembers everything, especially the events, feelings, and thoughts that are more intense than our everyday life experiences. These memories can be emotional, chemical, physical insults and injuries, or disease pathologies, but if they have not been processed, expressed, or released, they are held in the body. Thus they create a place that does not move as easily or function as well as it used to. These places can create the energy cysts we discussed earlier. The rest of the body has to move and work around these places, creating strain patterns throughout the body until, one day, our body cannot adapt to these any longer, and we begin to experience pain, illness, or dysfunction in body and mind.

TISSUE MEMORY IN FASCIA AND CELLS

Now we set our sights on tissue memory in fascia and individual cells. We will start with fascia, an extraordinary network of connective tissue that surrounds every single thing in our body, from the largest structures to the tiniest, even to every cell and the chromosomes inside the cell. It is a continuous sheet of delicate, fluid-filled fibers that change in structure in order to adapt to the function of that part of the body. It contains neurotransmitters, and electrolytes in solution, and it can contract and feel pain. It contains elastin that acts like an elastic band. If you take an elastic band and pull it out of shape and then let go of the pull, it will always return to its original shape and tension. Our fascia has this ability through its elastin. Where there is a pattern of tension or a place of immobility in our fascia, we can use our hands to facilitate the elastic memory and allow it to return to its original shape and tension. Part of this process may involve the work described above to facilitate the expression or release of some kind of memory in the tissue.

But we can be even more specific with our facilitation. We can work at a cellular level to facilitate helpful change. If our cells are not working well, nothing will work—no system in our body. Cells are the basic unit. Cells come together to make tissue; tissues work together to make organs; organs work together to make a body.

Once again, it is about safety. Even individual cells respond to danger in their environment, and here is what happens to them.

CELL DANGER RESPONSE

We are going to look at the cell danger response, relying on Robert K. Naviaux's research in "Metabolic Features of the Cell Danger Response.[19]"

The cell danger response is exactly what its name suggests. Our cells have an ancient response to threats or danger presented from different sources, such as viruses, bacteria, fungi, parasites, heat, salt, pH shock, UV, or chemical dangers. This ancient response is also activated by psychological trauma, particularly during childhood. The cells respond to physical and verbal violence. This response is triggered when threats to the safety and homeostasis of the cell overwhelm the capacity and resources of the cell to cope and maintain balance. If there is a mixed load of triggers, the impact is greater.

The cell danger response, once triggered, involves a cascade of changes. Once a harmful event is over, the cell will activate anti-inflammatory and restorative events, so it can heal. However, if there are many events and the response is activated for a long time, restoration and healing may not occur. The whole metabolism and the gut microbiota will be disturbed, many organ systems can be negatively affected, behavior can be changed, and chronic disease can result.

Deep within each cell, metabolic memory of past threats is stored. An awareness of the cell danger response allows us to see more clearly the potentially enormous impact of challenging experiences in early life on our body and mind, as shown in the Adverse Childhood Experience Study. It shows us how deep into the cells of our body these experiences can penetrate. It shows us how we are creatures that are primed through evolution to survive, to react, and to remember in our body any experience, whether emotional, physical, biological, or chemical, that threatens our safety. Further evidence of the long-term effects of childhood trauma and adversity is found in the work of Ehlert, "Enduring Psychobiological Effects of Childhood Adversity."[20] This research supports our belief that CranioSacral Therapy and SomatoEmotional Release can facilitate and activate the body-mind's self-healing responses to help an individual move forward from difficult life experiences.

This research into our cells' response to threat opens our eyes to the possible origins of a large range of chronic, developmental, degenerative, and autoimmune disorders that might include autism spectrum disorders, attention deficit hyperactivity disorder, asthma, sensitivities to gluten and other foods, Tourette's syndrome, mental health problems, post-traumatic stress disorder, epilepsy, traumatic brain injury, organ transplant biology, diabetes, cancer, Alzheimer's, Parkinson's, arthritis, and many, many others.

This research is talking about cells in general, but we can begin to ponder its application to the gut, the microbiome, and the enteric nervous system.

MITOCHONDRIA

Within our cells are the mitochondria, the organelles (tiny organs!) that act like a cell's digestive system. They take in nutrients, break them down, and create molecules full of energy. The connection between neurodegenerative episodes and infection in mitochondrial diseases was recognized by Edmonds and his researchers in their work titled "The Otolaryngological Manifestations of Mitochondrial Disease and the Risk of Neurodegeneration with Infection."[21] With the discovery that mitochondria are a key part of how our cells defend themselves from threats, and also a key to our immunity, this connection between neurological challenges and infection is beginning to be understood.

CELL DANGER RESPONSE, MITOCHONDRIAL DISEASE, AND THE ENTERIC NERVOUS SYSTEM

Let us take a moment to consider the connection between the cell danger response, the enteric nervous system, and mitochondrial disease and its influence on the health of our digestive system. We have just seen that the mitochondria and the cell danger response are part of the cell's defense system and our immunity.

There is some research into mitochondria, cell defense, and unexplained gastrointestinal symptoms, specifically that of Chapmen, et al., "Unexplained Gastrointestinal Symptoms: Think Mitochondrial Disease."[22]

Chronic stresses or threats to safety, which create chronic activation of the cell danger response and the mitochondria within the cell, change the physical habitat of the distant bowel and the availability of resources in the form of dietary nutrients. These changes occur because of the impact of chronic stresses and threats on the microbiome and the enteric nervous system. As we have already said, the gut bacteria, the microbiome, the enteric neurons, and the enteric glia talk to each other all the time.

Our metabolism is linked to our microbiome. A healthy gut microbiome means a healthy host, and a sick microbiome means a sick host. The collective metabolism of the microbiota and the human host influences long-term changes in gene expression by modifying the epigenetics of the DNA in our cells.[23]

These new understandings inform us about the consequences, shown above, both immediate and long-term, of adverse experience and emotional and mental stress on our digestive system.

CELLS SENSE THE RIGIDITY
OF THEIR ENVIRONMENT

Another new piece of research looks at how cells can sense the stiffness, or lack of tension, in the tissue around them. Researchers at the Max Planck Institute of Biochemistry in Martinsried have been able to show how cells sense the rigidity of their environment by measuring tiny mechanical forces and the influence of these forces on the cell.[24]

In the same way that we can feel whether we are lying on a soft blanket or hard rocks, our cells sense whether they are in a soft or rigid environment and can adapt accordingly. My question is, "Can cells function more optimally if their environment is not stiff and full of tension?"

I wonder, therefore, whether reducing the tension and patterns of restriction in the different layers of the gut might be a significant step in the direction of better gut function and health. It seems important for those in the Upledger CranioSacral Therapy world and other bodyworkers to have this knowledge. Think for a moment about stiff fascia, strain and tension patterns throughout the body, and, in particular, the gut tension patterns possibly holding the memory of the event that created this pattern.

MECHANICAL STRETCHING OF
CHROMATIN AND GENE EXPRESSION

There is still more to consider. External mechanical forces on cells can directly regulate gene expression.[25] This elegant study, showing the mechanical stretching of chromatin (the condensed DNA and protein mixture that makes chromosomes), identified the pathway that conveys an external mechanical force from the outside of the cell into the nucleus. The researchers stuck tiny magnetic beads to proteins attached to the external membranes of hamster cells. They managed to change the direction of the force the beads exerted, while, at the same time, keeping the amount of force consistent. They found that the external force directly caused regions of the chromatin in the nucleus to stretch out. By using advanced imaging techniques, the researchers found an increased transcription (the first stage of expression) of genes in the regions that were stretched.

Interestingly, the degree of stretching varied and, as a result, gene expression varied, depending on the direction of the force in relation to the cell's cytoskeleton, the internal framework of protein tubes that supports the cell. Researchers also discovered that some genes are activated by stretching of chromatin, and some are not.

While these studies are not specifically about the gut but about cells, we can clearly apply these principles to the cells in the gut and realize how mechanical forces influence the cells and gene expression. Tension patterns, surgeries, injuries, and infections or disease have many potential ways to influence the individual cells. The cell danger response, activity of mitochondria, rigidity of the environment of the cell, and mechanical stretching of chromatin, as well as the elastic memory in the elastin component of fascia, are ways already mentioned. There are very likely many more ways that have yet to be discovered.

In the world of Upledger CranioSacral Therapy, this raises some interesting questions. What makes genes ready to be activated by mechanical force? Is this another way in which, by working with fascia, we can connect into every cell and influence the chromatin and, therefore, gene expression? Can we change the way dysfunction in the body, and in particular the gut, is passed from one generation to the next through epigenetics? Can we reduce stretched areas of chromatin that are holding the memory of a mechanical force? As there are mechanical pathways for cells to change the gene expression and also to respond to the tension (or otherwise) of their environment, can we, with our hands and our intentions, use these and help shift them to create better health?

MICROGLIAL INVOLVEMENT IN CHRONIC PAIN

It seems that even molecules have a memory of synaptic activity. A new study at King's College, London, "Persistent Alterations in Microglial Enhancers in a Model of Chronic Pain,"[26] offers clues as to why chronic pain can persist, even when the injury that caused it has gone.

Researchers looked at microglia in mice. Microglia are a type of glial cell in the brain linked to the immune system and known to be important in generating persistent pain. Nerve damage in the mice was found to change epigenetic marks on some of the genes in their immune cells. The cells still behaved as normal, but the new epigenetic marks may mean they carry a "memory" of the initial injury.

Does chronic pain persist partly because of epigenetics? If the glial cells in the brain in the head are partly responsible for chronic pain that persists after the injury or dysfunction has gone, then do the gut's immune cells and the enteric glia in the second brain have a similar role in chronic gut pain?

MEMORY IN THE ENTERIC NERVOUS SYSTEM

Finally, there is an intriguing piece of research on memory in the enteric nervous system. Sustained Slow Postsynaptic Excitation (SSPE)[27] is small-intestine hypersensitivity and hyperreflexia caused when the autonomic nervous system overreacts to stimuli inside or outside the body. Even moderate stimulation of presynaptic inputs to the small intestine's intrinsic sensory neurons can result in substantially enhanced neuronal excitability that can outlast stimulation by several hours. SSPE may change activity in the long tube, resulting in functional bowel disorders.

To our knowledge, this is the only long-term change in the responsiveness of enteric neurons that has been discovered so far. Thus, it is a candidate mechanism for making our enteric nervous system overreactive.

GUT BACTERIA HAVE MEMORY TOO

There is one more thing to share about how our history becomes biologically ingrained in our body tissue. Turning our attention to the microbiota, the gut bacteria that work so closely with the enteric nervous system, it appears there is collective memory potential here.

Bacteria exposed to a moderate concentration of salt survive subsequent exposure to a higher concentration of salt better than if they had never been exposed to salt in this concentrated form before.[28] Interestingly, in individual cells, this effect does not last long. After just thirty minutes, the survival rate no longer depends on any previous exposure.

Two microbiologists discovered that when an entire population of the bacteria *Caulobacter crescentus,* found in freshwater, is observed under the microscope, the bacteria appear to develop a kind of collective memory. In populations exposed to a warning event, their rate of survival after a second exposure, as much as two hours after the warning, is better than in a population that has never been exposed. However, exposed populations may be more tolerant of future stress events, but sometimes they may be even more sensitive than populations with no previous exposure.[29]

✳

OUR BIOGRAPHY BECOMES OUR BIOLOGY!

There is a part of me sitting here that is concerned that you might feel a little—or more than a little—helpless when confronted with all these new studies on tissue memory. I am feeling a little of that too. It feels right now as if my gut—my long tube and my gastrointestinal tract—is some kind of museum, depicting my life story and possibly that of my parents and their parents. But do not despair; information is empowering. I have come from a dark place of almost complete dysfunction to a much better place where I can work, play, and continue to develop. Many, many people have made similar journeys.

Better understanding and awareness of how the gut works leads to more insights into the possible causal factors of the problems we find there. This sets the stage for facilitation of healing, probably through many paths, such as:

- reflecting on our emotional and mental stress levels both now and in the past
- addressing our lifestyle
- looking at the food we eat
- building our resources for responding to stress and challenge in our life
- recruiting help from bodyworkers, such as Upledger CranioSacral therapists, to destress our enteric nervous system, our autonomic nervous system, and our central nervous system and to release patterns of tension and restriction in the layers of the gut

- spending quiet moments listening to our body, and
- resolving issues still present in our bodies from the past—whether these are chemical, viral, bacterial, emotional, surgical, or possibly many other things

There are so many ways our life experience stays with and influences all of our physical selves that I wanted to write a poem to express some of this intensity.

Cell Memory

Synchronicity . . . Reflections . . . Flashes . . .
Stars in the belly
Stars in the head

Glial plasticity above and below
Learning, adapting
Reeling from stories
We told ourselves long ago

Afraid of the same characters
Being written into our lives again
Alert, hypersensitive
Listening

Whispers of old pain
In the villi
Echoing through the glial networks
Like a night wind in a tall forest
Catching the occasional word

Feeling the chill in the air
Walking our neuronal paths
Over and over again

Multigenerational trauma of all kinds, passing through the generations by epigenetic changes, as well as through molecular memory imprinting more of our history in our body-mind at a cellular level, are now receiving serious consideration in the medical community. This can be seen in research described earlier in this book.

For the purpose of this book, tissue memory in the gut seems to carry the trauma and challenges from our whole life, especially our early years and even our experiences in utero before birth.

◯ *And Breathe!*

If it is not too strange a concept for you to embrace, take a peaceful moment to talk to your cells sometime when you have your hands on your abdomen and are listening and connecting into your inner world. Notice what comes up into your awareness. You may be surprised at how much you can learn and help yourself by doing this. Our rational mind can only take us so far in our personal growth and understanding of our health and the causes of any disease process, chronic illness, and dysfunction in any part of our body-mind.

However, when we give ourselves some time to sit quietly, or walk in a peaceful place, we can listen more carefully to the messages our body might have for us. We can focus on a particular area that is troubling us and perhaps take our breath and our presence to that area. We are only limited by what we believe to be possible. If our intention is to listen to the cells in our small intestine for information, for example, we can do just that.

In my colleagues' experiences and in my own, all parts of our body love to be listened to and heard. Without any analyzing or problem solving, we can gently ask that area for information; we can ask how it is feeling; we can perhaps ask what happened to it to understand why it has this problem now. And then we can just sit with our awareness there and see what pops up. Learning to hear the softly spoken messages from our body can take patience and practice. It is very helpful to see an Upledger CranioSacral therapist who is highly skilled at facilitating this process from a very grounded and nonjudgmental place.

Case Story—Brian
Memory and the Body

Brian is an active, professional man in his forties. He presented to me with cluster headaches that had been part of his life since his mid-teens. Cluster headaches are known to be the most painful condition a human being can suffer. Women with this condition say they are worse than childbirth.

I evaluated him hands-on, after taking a full case history, which included a forceps delivery at birth, a concussion to the back of the head as a youngster, an appendectomy, and a repair for an inguinal hernia that involved three layers of mesh (Brian was a serious runner for much of his youth).

Interestingly, the area I was drawn to without any doubt or distraction was his gut. I asked him again if he has any digestive issues. He said no except he can be a bit flatulent. I began with my hands on his intestines and could immediately feel large amounts of tension there. My hands listened carefully, and I found myself working on the areas of scar tissue from Brian's two surgeries. Gradually and gently, both areas began to unwind and release, and the whole of the large and small intestine and the mesentery began to feel soft, mobile, and, to use Brian's own words, "to glide and slide again!"

This enabled me to release his neck and occipital cranial base and vagus nerve with comparative ease. He felt good after the treatment and very relaxed. This state of relaxation was unusual for him.

Sadly, his working life took over early in his treatment process. What I find interesting about Brian's story is the impact the surgeries had on his gut and the resulting impact the gut had on the rest of his system in causing the cluster headaches.

This Story's Message

Brian's story illustrates how clearly the Inner Physician will show us where to work on the body of the person who comes to us for treatment, even if there is no apparent "logical" connection.

9

Torn and Battered

My Heart's Clothes and the Complexities of Grief

Memory: Witnessing Violence

Oh, I am being watched. Sitting near me is a memory in the shadows. She looks bruised and battered, not from physical beatings, but from witnessing violence. Her skin seems gray, and a thin pale cotton dress hangs from her frame. Her shoulders are rounded and her chest concave. Her eyes are round and dark blue. I look deeply into her eyes and see there no joy or peace. Instead, I see a troubled and saddened young teenager. I think she is thirteen or fourteen years old. She is not really trying to get my attention, but her air of isolation and abandonment draws me in, and I walk toward her. As I approach her, I can feel my breath become shallow; my gut tightens, and my mood darkens.

Closer still, I peer into the spaces of her eyes and see and hear again scenes from our past, hers and mine. I see my mother screaming, Alfred driven to shout back. My ears used to be pounded by the noise. Now, as I stare down the long tunnel of her eyes, the sounds

130

are like an echo from the past but with a quality that suggests they are still going on. This is followed shortly afterward by the sound of intense, whole-body sobbing from my mother as she flings herself across her bed. How I hated to hear her despair and unhappiness. How I hated being in that house. I know now her emotional state made it impossible for her to nurture me and show me much love and affection, to find any kind of enjoyment in our relationship, but back then, I was confused and did not understand anything that was going on around me. At the same time, I was and am filled with a deep sadness and regret for me and for her. We were two trees in the same forest unable to move near to each other. Isolated. An opportunity lost forever.

The most frightening experiences were witnessing the physical violence from Pete—seeing the rage in his red, screwed-up face, spitting hateful words at her, as he hit her face and grabbed her by the wrist, twisting it and wrenching it behind her. Often, I would find her on the floor, bruised and feeling sorry for herself. This violence continued through the early years of their marriage after Alfred's death, until Pete was old; then the violence was purely verbal. Every attempt I made to help her move out and leave him was rejected, so I soon lost the small amount of compassion I had for her.

But the memory sitting before me has become a little older—perhaps seventeen—and is reminding me that I am missing the main story. Her eyes are full of this scene of violence and full of the moment I realized the final wall had dropped between my mother and me—the realization that even if I forgave her and Pete, the small broken remnants of our relationship were lying scattered all over the road where I found her lying. This story unfolds in front of the memory and me. It takes place when I am still living at home with my mother in our old Victorian house.

It was three days after Alfred died in the hospital. That is another story, Alfred's story. My mother had been having an affair with Pete for many months by that point. Alfred had just died in intensive care, where he had been for a week. I was in shock, and had not even been allowed to take a break from college. Instead I was told to go to school and just act as if nothing had happened. However bad the situation, no one ever talked about it, and we all behaved as if nothing had happened.

Pete came to our house and, as was often the case, he and my mother began to shout and scream at each other. I was in my room. The noise became louder and louder until I heard my mother open the front door and run out of the house. Pete ran after her, beat her up in the street, and left her on the road. I ran outside and helped her up, brought her inside the house, and sat her on the sofa. Immediately, Pete reappeared, red in the face, and shouted at me, "I *know* your father, not *knew* your father! He is still alive, and he doesn't want to know you!" My first thought was so clear. I thought my mother and Pete had put Alfred into an old people's home, so they could be together. I thought perhaps he was still alive. My hopes rose, as he was the only person who had never treated me badly. How telling it was that I assumed they were both more than capable of such a callous act. But any hopes were short lived. Pete battered his way out of the house. I was dazed, confused, and upset.

Looking into the eyes of this memory, I can see she is in freeze. Everything in her body is on pause, waiting for something.

My mother was sitting on the sofa, holding her bruised and swollen arm. She confirmed Pete's story. She had had an affair and I was the product of that affair, but she had never told me or Alfred. She was very upset, not on my behalf at all, but because she was worried I would not love her anymore. She had no concern for how this news might hurt me. My role was to reassure her, as was often the case, but this time, I found that almost impossible to do. I said nothing. I was left alone with all this. My system was overwhelmed.

A dull glaze has come down over the eyes of the memory as she crouches in a doorway somewhere in my mind, homeless and disconnected. I go and put my arms around her. Others of all ages and sizes are crowding around us now. I stay with them for a while. It is all I can do for now.

The Complexities of Grief

My mother was diagnosed with Parkinson's disease around twelve years before she died. Her gut had always been a problem for as long as I can remember. She was always constipated, and every night she took strong laxatives. From where I sit now, I am not surprised. She was probably ricocheting from fight or flight to freeze most of her life. She had no resources to deal with stress and no understanding of how to express her emotions in a mature way. She had clearly never learned any of this from her parents.

I know now that Parkinson's disease is often preceded by years of constipation. Like most neurodegenerative diseases, it begins in the gut. Why are we so surprised to discover that now? After all, Hippocrates, regarded as the founder of medicine as a rational science, said many centuries ago, "All disease begins in the gut."

Over the last ten years of her life, I watched her lose the ability to walk, to talk, to eat, and to make any facial expression. Her life became reduced to a bed downstairs; a hoist into a chair, where she ate soft purees offered by Pete; an endless stream of carers; a catheter, nappies; and then a hoist back into bed at night. She was on endless amounts of laxative and many other medications. I went through phases of feeling compassionate and helping my mother and Pete as much as I could and phases when I could barely bring myself to visit her. It was a horrible, slow, crumbling of a human being. I know she hated being helpless and so ill. It was sometimes surprising and a little heart-warming to see Pete making her food and feeding her. Other times, there were still signs of his temper—and her critical, brittle nature—when he had thrown the food against the wall of the living room and left it there to drip and then dry over the days and weeks that followed.

One day, when she was still able to talk and walk with a Zimmer frame (walker), she asked me to go upstairs with her. She slowly reached the Stannah stairlift, while I waited at the bottom of the stairs and then followed her up.

At the top of the stairs she faced the long journey along the corridor to her bedroom. Her feet were listening carefully for the occasional mixed message from her central nervous system; they moved awkwardly and in a broken rhythm as she struggled at the mercy of her broken brain. What do you do as the witness? Make conversation to pass the endless time the walk is taking, as if it is normal and there is no problem? Stand silently and stare at her? Offer occasional comments on her progress and how hard it must be? I found myself doing a mixture of all three, trying them out for size. None of them really fit the situation but somehow passed the time.

We reached her bedroom, and she maneuvered herself carefully into a controlled fall until she was sitting on the edge of her bed. I sat down beside her, relieved that the long walk was at an end. She sighed and rested her head on my shoulder. This was an unusual act for her. She said, "It would be better if I just died." The full weight of her suffering hit me—a suffering that stretched back through her whole life. An unexpected, uncontrollable wave of grief and compassion rose up through my body, and I burst out into sobs. I still feel an echo of the sadness from that time as I write. In that moment, we found ourselves—probably for the only time—in a shared, deep, aching grief for what had been in the past and for what had never been in the past, as well as a recognition that in the midst of that, there was love. Today I long for a chance to be in that place again, not because it would change anything, but because I could have an experience of our love.

One day, after several weeks of not feeling strong enough to visit her, I got a phone call from Pete to tell me my mother had had a stroke and it seemed serious. I decided to go and see her with both my children as soon as possible. We arrived and found her in bed. We all sat near her, and I could see she was falling backward down a long tunnel. Confusion and suffering were in her eyes. Remembering her looking so lost and unhappy is still so sad. She was unable to find a way through the damage in her brain toward the world. She seemed to recognize me, and I held her hand and told her it was alright and that I loved her. All the past seemed irrelevant at that moment, and I wanted her to know that none of that mattered anymore. My daughter reached across to hug her, but she was terrified and did not seem to know her; she lifted her birdlike arms up to defend herself from a perceived attack. This was upsetting to both of them. I felt so much sadness for my daughter—who had a better relationship with her than I ever had—that she was now unknown, a frightening stranger instead of a beloved granddaughter. We all sat close, not knowing what else to do. Eventually we left. I asked Pete to ring me and keep me updated. He rang a day or two later and relayed that the doctors said they did not know how long she had left, but that her passing did not seem imminent. The next day, Saturday morning, a Macmillan nurse* called me to say my mother died in the night. I was angry with Pete and felt he tried to keep us away. I would have liked to see her again.

---

*The UK term for a nurse specializing in palliative care.

Loss landed heavily on my heart when she died. Loss for any possibility of having the mother I would have liked; loss of the possibility of experiencing the feeling of safety at home; loss of the possibility of feeling nurtured and valued by her. That Saturday, two friends rescued me as I sobbed on the sofa. They brought me coffee and took me to see my mother's body. She was lying in a coffin, still and silent, no movement of her chest, no flickering of her eyes.

She was there and not there at the same time. It was all too late now, as I bent over and gently placed my lips on her forehead. It was cold and hard, and I wondered if my kiss would reach her somehow. I was contracted with grief and tears. Pale and stiff, her face was showing all of her despair and disappointment in life. I was just glad for her that it was over. I wished it had been different. The emptiness returned and filled me. I stood and stared at her. So this was the end.

Grieving for her was and is still complicated. I feel a mixture of emotions—relief from the pain of seeing her struggle with Parkinson's disease as it progressed rapidly the last few years; relief from having to be in the same room with her and Pete, where the past made being present with them so difficult; relief from never having to see Pete again; anger at the waste of her life, at the way she treated me, and at her selfish, immature emotionality; confusion at how to grieve for her and how to come to terms with the love I still feel for her, in spite of everything, a love that was never expressed or understood. Underneath all that, I know she loved me, but her love was tied up in the muddle of her life and could not find the air to breathe and be free. And above all, there is a sense of her despair in her life.

I am empty again. All words are gone for now. I am caught in this pause. My memories, like the homeless children they are, have left me and are walking along a dark street somewhere into the distance. I do not feel alone. I know some of you will have had similar or much worse experiences and that my story is not special. It is just a story, shared for the first time in the hope of holding some of you in a less lonely place. Much of it is written in the tissue of my body, especially my gut. Where is yours written?

At least it is a story my body has read to me, and I have listened. Together with help, facilitation, and most of all love from wonderful colleagues and close friends, a new story of safety and peace is being written in its place. For that I am eternally grateful. We are all authors in our lives. I sit here today wondering what new stories you might be writing and send you hope, joy, and peace.

Today, spring is nearly here, and the sun is shining clear and bright outside my window. There is a cold clarity in the air, a fresh expanded space to bring out all the potential born of the winter stillness. Where there is bright light, there is also shadow.

Memory: Freeze

My arm is gently touched by a young memory. She is about twelve years old. She has tiptoed out of the shadows to remind me of something. Her eyes are full of reproach. I turn at her touch and look into her eyes with confusion. What is she trying to tell me? She pulls my head down toward hers and whispers in my ear, "You have forgotten to talk about Alfred and everything he did for you. He tried his best. And you have forgotten to tell everyone how you went into a deep state of freeze when he died, that a part of you stayed frozen for around twenty years. Have you forgotten that you, like your mum, were always constipated for many years while your gut was held in pause?"

I tell her I have not forgotten any of this and that I will tell her story next. So here it is.

Alfred, as you probably remember, was the man my mother was married to and who I thought was my father for many years. He was twenty years older than she was and quite ill for as long as I can remember—first with tuberculosis scarring, which meant he had to have most of one lung removed; then glaucoma, which took away his ability to read; and finally he had a stroke, which left him confused and uncertain. In his younger days, before I was born, he was a brilliant history teacher with an incredible mind and ability to connect with his students. Before this, he was a singer with a huge, rich bass voice, even though he was not that tall and was very slender. He also wrote children's stories and poetry. It would have been wonderful to know him before he was so old and ill. But I have some of his poems and his books. He was always kind to me, apart from his attempts to get me to side with him after the many loud arguments with my mother, and he never hit me. He made me toast or toasted crumpets when I came home from school. (He was retired, and my mother worked full time.) He did not have the strength to do very much. I remember how unhappy he was over the last few years of his life.

It was also Alfred who saw my suffering in the family and suggested I join a drama group. Old and ill as he was, he often took me there on the bus and repeated the journey to pick me up afterward. Eventually, Alfred was not able to do this, so I went alone. This introduction to and immersion in the performing arts was another saving grace in my life and has remained with me to this day. The benefits were huge, and twice per week, I could be someone else, explore another life, explore emotional experience in a safe way, and find relief for a while from my own. Most of all, I could explore relationships.

I could see his life had little joy remaining and soon it was to be over. My mother was away on holiday, and Alfred and I were at home. I was seventeen years old. It was peaceful—no arguments, shouting, or sobbing. I was probably upstairs in my bedroom, where I spent so much time alone. I went downstairs and saw him in his chair. But something was wrong. I noticed Alfred was very quiet and pale. He was sitting in the living room in the chair he spent so much time in, staring into space. (Unable to read, he watched a lot of TV.) Disappointment and despair were etched on his thin face. He looked at me, said he was in a lot of pain, and asked if I would call the doctor. He had taken painkillers, but his gut was tied up in a continuously agonizing cramp. I called our general practitioner, and he came quickly. He examined Alfred and called for an ambulance, then asked me to put a bag together with pajamas and everything he might need, as he would have to go into the hospital.

I quickly collected his things, the ambulance arrived, and he was carried out on a sitting-up stretcher. I had just passed my driving test and followed the ambulance to the hospital in the battered, old mini my mother had left at home.

I waited and waited through the early hours of the morning. I do not remember feeling any emotion. I felt held in a strange, disconnected moment. Now I know this was freeze. Eventually I was taken to see Alfred. He looked gray. The doctors told me his gut was twisted, and they would need to operate the next day. I tried to reassure him that everything would be okay, and I left to drive home. It was somewhere near dawn. I went to bed alone in our old Victorian house, feeling very scared. Every sound made me jump, and sleep was not my friend. I felt very unsafe.

The next day is unclear in my memory, sitting here so many years later. I think I called the hospital, and they asked me to call my mother and bring her home. I am not sure I realized how serious this was. She came home later that day and together we went to see Alfred in the hospital after the surgery. We went every day for a week. Things had not gone well during surgery, and he was in intensive care. Those visits are still so clear in my memory—standing still, watching him lying in bed. The sound score to our visits was a mechanical symphony of machines pumping air in and out of his lungs, dripping fluids into each hand, monitoring every heartbeat. Underneath this score was a silent drip of blood from each hand to the floor. There were too many tubes, too many struggles. How unlike himself he looked. His face, somehow smaller, was almost mask-like; his eyes sunk into his skull. I searched his face for the only person who had been kind to me, in spite of his illness and lack of strength. I could not find him there. I think he had taken this opportunity to leave a life that had nothing left for him. There was little to bring him back. Every day, as I climbed the stairs and walked the long corridors to where he—or some residue of him—lay, my legs would ache more and more. My heart was numb. I have no memory of my mother at this time—how she looked, what she said or felt. My instinct is that it was not much. She'd had no love left for Alfred for many years.

The hospital called around eight o'clock in the morning, as I was getting ready to go to the Further Education College, where I was doing a course. Alfred had died in the night. I stood very still, waiting for something unknown. My mother told me to go to college as usual. I did not argue. I felt numb, and now I was excluded from any process of grief.

That something stayed unknown for many years. My friends at college asked me how my father was. I had told them he was in the hospital. I remember clearly being so embarrassed to say he had died. They were shocked at my emotionless presence, not liking to ask straight out why I was not at home. I had to be emotionless to be there at all. Freeze was the only place for me. That day, and the days that followed, rode over my unspoken feelings like horses galloping across my heart. Even so, my heart somehow remained mysteriously untouched by the rhythmic trampling of their hooves. This experience was all too familiar, at once distant and close.

It was to be many years, around twenty-five years later, that my body memory took me back to that time during a CranioSacral Therapy session. Once again, I was standing silent and overwhelmed in the intensive care unit, watching the slow drip of blood from an old man's birdlike hand to the floor. This time, I became aware of the restriction in my abdomen and in my chest, holding all my grief inside. The difference now was that I was supported by a group of CranioSacral therapists who created such a safe place for me that the tension crumbled, and I melted into a river of tears, finally grieving for the one kind adult in my life. The relief this brought to my body was enormous and welcome, as I was no longer being held in a pattern of chronic back pain and constipation. It was the beginning of a freedom and transformation in my life. I am forever grateful.

Looking back now, it feels as if my mesentery may have been involved in linking and gripping my back and my gut, and I wonder about the complex interaction between the dorsal vagal complex, the mesentery, the gut, and life.

Postscript

I have come back to this chapter on grief a month later. Yesterday, I learned that my half-brother, John, died early in the morning after a long battle with cancer. I listened to the voicemail on my phone between seeing patients in my clinic. I had to listen twice. I felt an immediate ache and heavy tension in my solar plexus, in my gut, and for a few moments was unsure that I could continue to work with the patients still to come. I decided I could; after all, burying feelings was once the norm for me. It turned out that I am not so adept at this anymore, and waves of sadness and loss washed over me all afternoon. John was the son of my mother and Alfred. He was very clever and was sent to expensive schools all through his life, ending up at Oxford University. Most of these were boarding schools, so he was not really present in my life while I was growing up. He escaped most of the violence and misery that permeated life in our house. I always felt stupid compared to him.

Sitting here today, the day after, I am full of sadness for my family. John's death has brought back so much of the many losses sharply and painfully into my heart and life. I wish so many things had been different for all of us. I am holding on to a conversation I had with him on the phone just over a month ago, the first in a long time, in which we made a new connection and talked about some of the past from our different perspectives. He was so happy to hear what I was doing with my life and that I had remarried. I was learning what an amazing person and teacher he was, and I was wanting to learn more. He did not let me know how very ill he was. We agreed to stay in touch, and oddly, it was today that I had planned to call—a day too late, as it turned out. I regret that deeply. The night before his death, I was awake much of the night, not really knowing why, feeling wobbly and nauseous. Now I know why. Last night and today, my gut was full of grief and pain—sore, overactive, nauseous, exhausted—so many memories activated. The biggest emotion there is loss and the impossibility of changing that loss. The entering of the outside world into me seems harsh and almost unbearable today. I have no anger; just a feeling of so much love for my mother, Alfred, and John that was somehow impossible for any of us to experience in the confusion of our lives together. What to do with this? I don't know.

Perhaps these few words I gathered together in a poem for John just after I heard of his death will resonate with some of you who are in the midst of complex grieving. I am there with you.

For My Brother

Tears and stumbling words
Fall echoing
Into the empty space

between

us

too late. You have already left.
I lift my eyes to see you. But death has robbed
me of that tender view.

Sorrow and regret stand beside me now

unwelcome new companions

The space is still empty

10

Peering down
the Microscope

SEROTONIN AND THE GUT

To understand where our gut feelings come from, I think it is helpful to look in detail at the different cells and systems in place there that cocreate much of our emotional and physical health.

It is time to be fascinated by the tiny things again! Did you know you have micromuffins in your gut? That is my nickname for the fascinating enterochromaffin cells that are found in specific locations throughout the gastrointestinal tract, mostly in the small intestine, colon, and appendix. In the small intestine, they are in the loose, sponge-like layer we looked at called the lamina propria, and they particularly like the crypts between the intestinal villi.

Enterochromaffin cells manufacture and store at least 90 percent of the body's serotonin.[30] Serotonin made in the gut naturally calms the digestive system, stimulates peristalsis, and is deeply involved in our digestion. But once this work is done, serotonin is also involved in our feeling of well-being.

I wonder about the impact of the popular family of selective serotonin reuptake inhibitor (SSRI) antidepressants on the gut.

SSRIs are believed to ease depression by enhancing levels of available serotonin in the brain. But the brain in the head contains only 5–10 percent of our serotonin.

What happens to our enteric nervous system and microbiome when there is free serotonin in the gut? Low levels of serotonin in the brain and the gut are associated with depression and with constipation. These drugs divert supplies of serotonin from their natural receptors in the gut and thus can create anxiety, alter sleep patterns, and cause sexual dysfunction. Does this help explain why users of SSRIs often experience nausea, constipation, diarrhea, fluctuations in appetite, and altered sleep patterns? The use of SSRIs can upset the delicate balance required in the digestive system.

Interestingly, the enterochromaffin cells need input from some particular strains of gut bacteria to achieve optimum serotonin-production levels. When these bacteria are missing, there is a staggering reduction in the serotonin they can make—about 60 percent less.[31]

OTHER PHARMACEUTICALS AND THE GUT

Serotonin is fat-soluble and can penetrate the gut wall. But what about all the other fat-soluble drugs that can penetrate the gut wall, such as sleeping pills and tranquilizers?

The gut naturally produces benzodiazepines to keep the natural state of calm that is necessary for proper functioning. GABA receptors for artificial benzodiazepines and sleeping pills are also in the gut and also can depress gut movement, which can lead to constipation. Filling the GABA receptors with tranquilizers and sleeping pills throws this natural function out of balance and can create chronic gut issues. Long-term use of medications that target GABA receptors place stress on the body.

In many ways, the connection between stress and the gut may be the most visible gut-brain connection. Chronic stress can result in indigestion, constipation, ulcers, and a host of uncomfortable symptoms, including colon spasms.

HOW ENTEROCHROMAFFIN CELLS COMMUNICATE

Coming back to the enterochromaffin cells, let's next consider their potential role in communication with both the gut and the brain.

Most enterochromaffin cells communicate with the lumen through the microvilli (protrusions) and are referred to as "open." Some of the enterochromaffin cells do not protrude into the lumen and are subsequently referred to as "closed." Enterochromaffin cells typically extend down to the basal lamina (part of the basement membrane we explored in an earlier chapter). Tissue beneath enterochromaffin cells typically contains many fenestrated capillaries that allow some proteins and small molecules to come through their walls, lymph vessels, and small unmyelinated nerve fibers. Serotonin secreted from the enterochromaffin cells can either be taken up into residing capillary vessels (transported in the blood by platelets) or act on nerve synaptic terminals, thus modulating neuronal activity.

Enterochromaffin cells respond to mechanical and sensory events in the lumen. Most of these cells protrude into the lumen and also have extensions into the layers of tissue beneath them. They are pleomorphic, which means they can alter their size and shape in response to their environment. They control communication between the gut lumen and the nervous system. They are stimulated by nutrients as well as by tastants, which create a perception of flavor, and they respond by secreting hormones that are powerful influences on our appetite.

Enterochromaffin cells talk to enteric neurons and enteric glia—necessarily because the enteric neurons and enteric glia do not reach into the lumen. As they are important bidirectional transducers (they change a signal in one form of energy into another form of energy), they can then modulate the activity of enteric neurons. The enterochromaffin cells act as translators (fig. 7). They control communication between the gut lumen and the nervous system.

They are also an important part of the microbiota-gut-brain axis (fig. 8; p. 149) as they are affected by the gut bacteria and talk to the enteric neurons and enteric glia.

You might guess that more enterochromaffin cells means more serotonin production and therefore more happiness. But this is clearly not the case in the gut, where too much serotonin stimulates rapid and frequent peristalsis. Abnormal, overabundant populations of

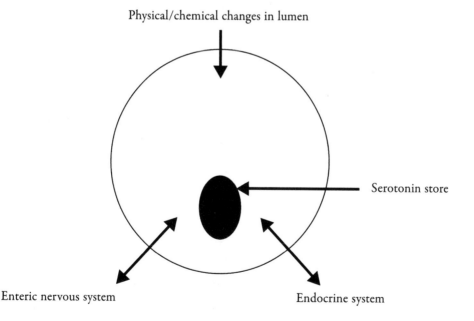

Physical/chemical changes in lumen

Serotonin store

Enteric nervous system

Endocrine system

Figure 7. Enterochromaffin cell as a bi-directional transducer that can talk to enteric neurons as well as enteric glia.

enterochromaffin cells are associated with irritable bowel syndrome and other bowel dysfunctional diseases. This research appears in an article titled "Is Irritable Bowel Syndrome an Organic Disorder?"[32] And there is more research such as the article "Serotonin and GI Disorders: An Update on Clinical and Experimental Studies."[33] A larger number of enterochromaffin cells than normal is associated with diarrhea and a decreased number with constipation. Perhaps there is an ideal level of serotonin for digestion and emotional well-being to be functional and stable?

ENTERIC GLIAL CELLS

The enteric glial cells turn out to be a vital part of nurturing the enteroendocrine cells.[34] The research shows a physical relationship between enteric glial cells and enteroendocrine cells, such as enterochromaffin cells, with the glial cells escorting the enteroendocrine cells.

We have seen already that we have conversations inside us between enteric glia, enterochromaffin cells, and enteric neurons. And, of course, these conversations include the enteric microbiota. It is becoming clearer that chronic stress and trauma disrupt the smooth interactions between these cells and create functional and inflammatory bowel disorders as well as mental health issues (if you separate the mind from the body in this way), such as anorexia, bulimia, anxiety, depression, schizophrenia, post-traumatic stress disorder, and, of course, my idea of Post-Traumatic Gut Disorder.

While we have the microscope out, we can explore the wide range of functions and activities of our enteric glia and a specialized subtype of enteric glia called the mucosal enteric glial cells.

Enteric glial cells are a unique class of peripheral cells within the gastrointestinal tract. Major populations of enteric glia are found packed tightly around the neurons, in enteric ganglia, and in the myenteric and submucosal plexus of the enteric nervous system.

They are also found outside the enteric nervous system, within the circular muscle and the lamina propria of the mucosa, and extend their reach to the end of every single villus protruding into the lumen. There are probably different types of glia in the gut that have differing functions, just as there are in the brain in the head. We do not have all these categories sorted out yet! But they seem to be involved in almost every gut function including

Microbiota-Gut-Brain Axis

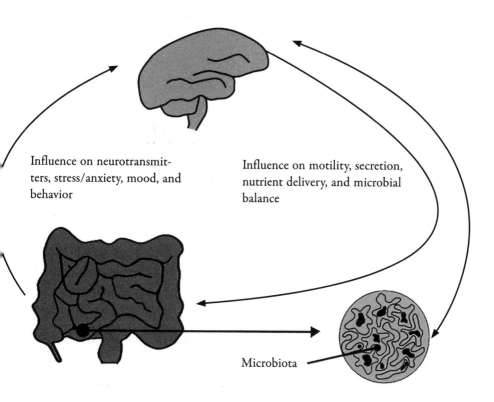

Influence on neurotransmitters, stress/anxiety, mood, and behavior

Influence on motility, secretion, nutrient delivery, and microbial balance

Microbiota

Figure 8. The microbiota-gut-brain axis facilitates important conversations between the gut bacteria (the microbiota), the gut and its enteric nervous system, and the brain in the head.

movement and secretion of mucus. With the immune system, they also defend the body from attack.

Many enteric glial cells are little cells: they are similar to the astrocytes with their star-like appearance but not quite the same, nor are they exactly like Schwann cells, the glial cells of the peripheral nervous system. The little, star-like enteric glial cells surround nerve processes in the mucosa, thereby making a close connection with the epithelial cells (more about both of those soon), while another population wraps around neuronal cell bodies in the two plexuses.

Until recently, neurons were thought of as the only active cells in the enteric nervous system. Gut function was thought to be coordinated by how neurons talk to one another. Now, it is known that the enteric glia do much more than provide a supportive network for neurons; they have been observed to "listen" to the "conversations" between neurons as research shows us "imaging neuron-glia interactions in the enteric nervous system."[35] A major focus of research is to find out how the glia cells influence these conversations and, as a result, influence gut function as seen in the article "Emerging Roles for Enteric Glia in Gastrointestinal Disorders."[36]

The path of understanding is very similar to the one already trodden in the central nervous system and our understanding of glia cells there. We know that glia cells in the central nervous system support every neuron and every synapse, and they are activated by neuronal activity as well as activate it. Glial cells in the central nervous system are involved in our creativity, memory, and learning. Neurons in the central nervous system cannot survive without glia cells. My esteemed colleague Tad Wanveer has written the book *Brain Stars* referenced earlier, which is all about the wonderful work of central nervous system glial cells.

Enteric glial cells actively process and integrate information between enteric neurons and enteroendocrine cells, as well as form part of the intestinal epithelial barrier. They work in networks, and they often join their cells together. This idea is supported by the description of calcium waves traveling in a wavelike fashion between cultured enteric glial cells after mechanical or chemical stimulation of an individual glial cell. Research from the National Institutes of Health[37] shows us more about how enteric glial cells are implicated increasingly in inflammatory bowel disease.

Enteric glial cells are also activated by synaptic stimulation from neurons,[38] suggesting an active role in conversations between neurons, but the precise role is currently unclear.

Enteric glial cells are actively involved in enteric neuroplasticity. Our enteric nervous system can change and adapt just as our central nervous system can and does. Incredibly, enteric glial cells have given rise to neurons in vivo in response to chemical injury to the enteric ganglia. There is no inherent way to create new neurons in the adult gut, but it seems that enteric glial cells still have some potential to do this if there is an injury.[39] Interestingly, this is mirroring new insights into neurogenesis in the brain, which was also believed to be incapable of producing new neurons. The clinical implications are huge and positive. How might CranioSacral therapists influence this potential?

Enteric glial cells help maintain and repair the intestinal epithelial barrier that separates the lumen from the body. When enteric glial cells are reduced in numbers, the barrier's tight junctions and mucous layer are disrupted.[40] This creates vulnerable areas where noxious molecules, viruses, and other inappropriate substances can penetrate the barrier, activate our immune system, and find their way into the blood circulation.

Enteric glial cells are also part of the blood-enteric barrier. Enteric glial cells have expanded end feet, just as the astrocytes do in the brain, where they are an important part of the blood-brain barrier. The blood-enteric barrier protects the enteric neurons from potentially harmful extra ganglionic substances and protects the blood from potentially harmful bacteria and viruses. I will share more about both these barriers below.

Enteric glial cells are affected by stress,[41] which negatively affects the intestinal epithelial barrier above everything else. Does this mean there could be a loss of enteric glia with stress, and that loss of enteric glia impacts on the barrier? Or does it mean that when stress affects the barrier, enteric glia are lost? Whichever direction it goes, stress often results in intestinal inflammation and disruption of the epithelial barrier. It turns out that people with severe constipation or inflammation in the gut do have decreased numbers of enteric glia. Remember they also have fewer "muffins" (enterochromaffin cells).

In addition to these roles, enteric glial cells interact with lymphocytes and respond actively to inflammation, bringing immune cells to the enteric nervous system. They help the immune system within the gut to make an appropriate response to any challenges. Think about irritable bowel syndrome, Crohn's disease, and inflammatory bowel disease, to name just a few issues.

I am wondering if their immune response has any similarities to the microglia, the little glial cells in the brain that respond to infection and injury.

This all makes it likely that enteric glia may serve as a link between the nervous and immune systems of the gut. And when you consider that 70 percent of our immune system is in the gut, this connection is very important to our health (fig. 9).

MUCOSAL ENTERIC GLIAL CELLS

We are going to meet one more fascinating specialist subtype of enteric glia, the mucosal enteric glial cells (mEGCs), which are found in the lamina propria. The cellular microenvironment of mEGCs

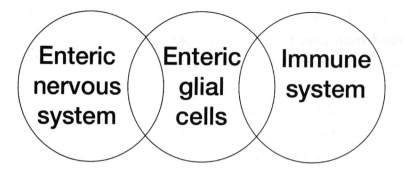

Figure 9. Enteric glial cells are a link between the enteric nervous system and the immune system mucosal enteric glial cells.

in the lamina propria is unique, as the lamina propria is only one cell away from the rich microbiome in the intestinal lumen. These mEGCs are therefore at the forefront of our contact with the outside world, the lumen, and all the diverse cells found in the lamina propria.

The mEGCs are extensively branched, and their processes are known to contact immune cells, enteric neurons, enteroendocrine cells (like enterochromaffin cells), and blood vessels. In other words, the mEGCs are perfectly placed to integrate intercellular signaling. They talk to and link the work of the immune system, the endocrine system, and the enteric neurons in the gut, which is fascinating and very clever.

Interestingly, it seems the microbiota is essential for normal mEGC development.[42]

THE INTESTINAL EPITHELIAL BARRIER

All this little stuff is the basis of all the big stuff. A healthy gut is fundamental to a healthy life. It is a place where we are exposed to the external world and vulnerable to invasion from viruses, fungi, and bacteria that might not be good for us. It is also a place impacted by stress and emotional challenge as well as the impacts of carrying our history. It appears we have an incredible system to help keep the bad guys out and let the good guys in. Let me introduce you to its rich diversity.

First, let us look in detail at the innermost layers of the long tube—the small intestine in particular—where our maximum absorption of nutrients takes place. We will start from the lumen (again, that's the space in the middle of the tube).

We meet our intestinal epithelial barrier first, which has two parts: intrinsic and extrinsic. The intrinsic part of the barrier creates the anatomical and immunological barrier between the lumen, the external world, and our internal world. Remember that above the submucosa and the submucosal plexus, we have the lamina propria mucosae, which leads us to the epithelial layer that is composed of a single layer of intestinal epithelial cells. This is our intrinsic barrier—a single layer of cells!

The lamina propria and epithelial layer push together to create folds, called plicae circulares, and all along the edge are villi that protrude into the lumen. These folds increase the surface area of the small intestine. Recall that villi are finger-like projections that wave the food along in rhythm with peristalsis in the small intestine. The villi massively increase the surface area for absorption—approximately thirtyfold. The tiny microvilli, rising like a brush border on the surface of each epithelial cell, increase it by approximately a further six-hundred-fold. Together they create an incredibly efficient diffusion system. There are no villi in the large intestine, which is primarily for elimination rather than absorption of nutrients.

There is a very fast rate of cell death and regeneration of the epithelium—every four to five days. In each and every villus, there is a capillary bed and lymphatic duct. In between each villus is a dip, called a crypt, that generates new epithelial cells from stem cells and pushes them up to repair the epithelial layer. The rapid cell death leaves behind lots of dead cell bodies. Macrophages take these in the lamina propria, and the lymphatic system carries away the dead cell bodies. The positive aspect of this rapid cell death and regeneration is that we have the potential to heal and restore our epithelium to good function.

The epithelial layer is thin in order to create a short diffusion pathway. It is made up of a variety of cells—secretory cells, endocrine cells, and absorptive epithelial cells—that take up the nutrients from the lumen into the bloodstream. It is a two-way interface between the many different populations of luminal microbes and the immune cells of the lamina propria underneath.

This barrier is created by tight junctions in between the cells, which control what can get through these tight spaces. If the tight junction barrier is disrupted, toxic molecules from the lumen can penetrate the barrier, upsetting the immune system in the lamina propria and creating inflammation. This can be the beginning of intestinal and systemic diseases. These toxic molecules also have unimpeded access to systemic blood circulation (and can occasionally reach the blood-brain barrier and sometimes go through it).

Secreted over the top of this delicate barrier is a thin layer of mucus, and mucus softens shear stresses on the epithelium. The unwanted bacteria stick to the mucous layer, which helps to prevent their getting into the epithelium. The stickiness clumps the bacteria together and speeds up the process of clearing them away.

Differences in the Epithelial Layer in the Duodenum and Stomach

If we look further up the long tube to the duodenum of the small intestine and stomach, we see that the gastric and duodenal epithelial cells secrete bicarbonate ions that keep the pH neutral along the epithelial layer in very acidic conditions. In addition, these secretions, mucus in the jejunum and ileum of the small intestine and mucus plus bicarbonate ions in the duodenum and stomach, create the extrinsic part of the intestinal epithelial barrier.

The other parts of the mucosa, the basement membrane and lamina propria, support the barrier and, together with the barrier, create the immune system in the gut. And remember, this comprises 70 percent of our whole immune system!

Support from the Basement Membrane

I described the basement membrane earlier when we were looking at the layers of the small intestine. Here it seems important to underline how important the basement membrane is in terms of its support of the barrier, as it separates the epithelium from the underlying tissue (the lamina propria), as well as influences the epithelial cells by controlling their shape, gene expression, adhesion, migration, proliferation, and cell death.

In my clinical practice, I often find strain patterns in this basement membrane and find in its release great benefit to the person I am treating.

Support from the Lamina Propria

The lamina propria is a key place for immune response as it is full of immune cells as well as macrophages that eat up and dispose of the dead cells from the delicate, thin epithelial layer that forms the barrier above. The lamina propria is also a part of our defense from invading pathogens.

Because it can contract, the lamina propria helps pull tissue together to heal wounds. It also contributes massively to inflammation and wound healing responses by releasing cytokines and chemokines in response to stress—emotional, mental, mechanical, or chemical.

It provides support and nutrition to the epithelium as well as a way of binding its irregular surface to its underlying tissue, the muscularis mucosae that separate the lamina propria from the submucosa.

In my clinical practice, I often work specifically with my intention in the lamina propria, feeling for strain patterns, facilitating its own stories, and perhaps dialoguing with the cells to find out more about their status and function.

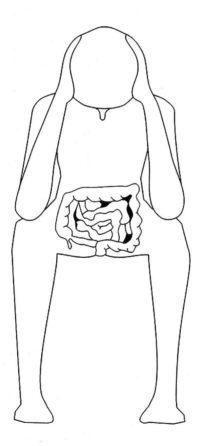

Figure 10. Mental and emotional health are
fundamentally connected to a healthy gut.

Together, all the layers of the small intestine are central to the health of our gut and therefore to our whole body-mind system. Too often regarded in a purely digestive capacity, the impact of damage or dysfunction in any of the layers on our immune health, our neurological health, our mental health, and our emotional health is unbounded.

Blood-Enteric Barrier

As we have noted above, the enteric glia are a big part of the intestinal epithelial barrier. There is a second barrier that works in concert with the intestinal epithelial barrier. Let's take a few moments to look at the comparatively recent discovery of this second barrier, which researchers Spadoni et al.[43] call the gut-vascular barrier (or GVB) and which I call the blood-enteric barrier.

These researchers found that if unwanted bacteria manage to enter the body, they tend to end up in the lymph nodes and not in the blood vessels near the small intestine. The nutrients we absorb enter the blood vessels next to the small intestine and go to the liver through the hepatic portal vein. The researchers could not find any of the unwanted bacteria in the liver. Their research discovered the blood-enteric barrier that prevents unwanted bacteria from getting into the blood vessels near the intestine along with the nutrients being absorbed.

Just a reminder to me, to all of us, that the biggest cause of disruption and damage to the intestinal epithelial barrier, and I imagine possibly to the newly found blood-enteric barrier, is stress, which comes in many forms and always comes along with illness and trauma. Just look at the research in *Nature* titled "Chronic Stress and Intestinal Barrier Dysfunction."[44]

GUT ENVIRONMENT: BALANCE OF INFLAMMATION AND REPAIR

The gut environment is a delicate balance of inflammation and repair. Sometimes the influences overwhelm the immune defenses, or the immune system overreacts, creating a chronic inflammatory environment. An overburdened immune system will not be able to prevent damage to the intestinal epithelial barrier that protects the body and the organs.

Once noxious bacteria get past the gut barrier, the body or somatic immune system can be easily overwhelmed. When the immune system cannot keep up with the chronic invasion, symptoms begin to develop. A compromised barrier is the very beginning of many symptoms, syndromes, and diseases—autoimmune conditions, headaches, insomnia, Lyme disease, anxiety, depression, neuroses, schizophrenia, myalgic encephalomyelitis, Parkinson's, multiple sclerosis, and many more.

To summarize, healthy and numerous enteric glial cells are vital to the nurture, support, and repair of the barrier. When they are depleted, the tight junctions of the barrier are disrupted, as is the mucosal layer, and this leads to inflammation. These effects of glial ablation on the mucosal barrier functions are not always communicated by enteric nerves but show a direct interaction between enteric glia and epithelial cells. This direct interaction further underlines the importance of our enteric glial cells to a healthy system.

Gut Barrier Repair

So how does the intestinal epithelial barrier repair after an invasion? Following disruption, the critical first task is to cover the denuded area and reestablish the intrinsic barrier. The rapid repair of the epithelium is achieved by a process called restitution. This is when epithelial cells adjacent to the vulnerable area flatten and migrate over the exposed basement membrane. In the small intestine, this process is aided by a rapid contraction and shortening of the affected villi, which reduces the area of the basement membrane that must be covered.

Although restitution provides a quick way of covering any defect in the barrier, it does not create more epithelial cells; the area, while protected, is not physiologically functional. The intestinal permeability can be repaired by first removing the source of inflammation and then nourishing the epithelial cells, so they can replicate and make new tight junctions. Full healing requires that the epithelial cells on the margins of the defect multiply and migrate into the damaged area to rebuild the normal cellular architecture and re-create normal function. Once the gut barrier is restored, the somatic immune system will be able to rebalance itself and hyperactivity will subside. Of course, with trauma and chronic stress, it is not always simple or even possible to remove the source of inflammation and damage. It will very likely require attention to diet, attention to emotional and mental stresses and stories in the gut, lifestyle changes, exercise, building resilience, and so on.

COMPARING THE BARRIERS

Comparing the barriers in the gut with the blood-brain barrier, as researchers at the University of California and the European Institute of Oncology in Milan, Italy, have been,[45] is proving interesting and enlightening. I have often found in my clinical practice that if the person I am working with has an issue in one of these barriers, it feels as if they also have an issue in the other. They seem to have influence on each other, not surprisingly perhaps. Let us take a few minutes to compare them in terms of cells, connections, and pathways.

Why would we compare the barriers? Comparison of the barriers will help us have a better understanding of many diseases. Each barrier undergoes similar changes during pathological inflammation. For example, food molecules that pass through the intestinal epithelial barrier into the bloodstream can then act on the blood-brain barrier, and the central nervous system molecules that leave the brain can access the intestinal epithelial barrier. Thus it is important not only to consider each barrier in isolation, but in the context of the whole organism, to realize the barriers work together to maintain homeostasis and that the function of each barrier may influence the other.

Both barriers provide defense in very different environments, but there are many similarities in action. In both cases, there is a physical barrier formed by a layer of cells that tightly controls the movement of ions, molecules, and cells between two tissue spaces. These barrier cells have a dynamic interaction with many different kinds of cells and with a different array of immune cells that keep watch over the physical barrier and provide adaptive immunity.

The intestinal epithelial barrier interacts with the microbiota and innocuous food antigens to protect against invading pathogens. In a way, it is our first defense against the world. The associated blood-enteric barrier protects the enteric nervous system from unwanted invaders.

The blood-brain barrier is formed by blood vessels of the central nervous system. In most tissues, blood vessels are leaky, allowing free flow of molecules and ions from blood into tissue. But in the central nervous system, blood vessels tightly restrict the flow of blood-borne ions and other molecules from entering the neural tissue. The blood-brain barrier is an important secondary barrier after the gut barrier to protect central nervous tissue that will fail to regenerate after injury and disease.

Researchers are finding remarkable similarities of barrier properties, so studies of one barrier may provide important insight into the other barrier. As mentioned, both barriers have a physical barrier formed by a cellular layer that tightly regulates the movement of ions, molecules, and cells between two different kinds of tissue; both barriers interact with many different immune cells that are protecting the barriers; and both barriers have glial cells in close contact with them that are involved in the structure and function of each barrier. Astrocytes are an important part of the blood-brain barrier, and the enteric glial cells, which are very similar to astrocytes, are part of the intestinal epithelial barrier.

There are also several differences between the two barriers. The first difference is that the intestinal epithelial barrier is constantly exposed to the microbiota and the lumen, so it is equipped, as we have already noted, with a mucous layer to protect us from the external world by physically separating microbiota from epithelial barrier. The blood-brain barrier is not exposed to the microbiota and so does not have a mucous layer; instead it has a complex glycocalyx layer, a highly hydrated, fibrous meshwork of carbohydrates that projects out and covers the membrane of endothelial cells, many bacteria, and other cells. The scientific literature suggests that this glycocalyx layer acts as a molecular sieve to block interaction of large blood-borne molecules.[46] The gut barrier protects us from external hazards, whereas the blood-brain barrier protects the central nervous system from hazards that are within the organism already. But central nervous system endothelial cells resemble epithelial cells, in that they are also held together by tight junctions.

Another difference is that each barrier has different cell type origins. In the gut the epithelial cells are endodermal* in origin, whereas in the central nervous system, the endothelial cells are mesodermal† in origin.

We have seen how the barriers are controlled by conversations between barrier cells and glial cells that are, of course, connected with the enteric nervous system and the central nervous system. This neural coupling may provide a unique mechanism for these barriers to talk to each other. We can ponder again our list of neuro-degenerative diseases, such as Alzheimer's, dementia, ME, multiple sclerosis, brain tumors, stroke, autism spectrum disorder, and mental and emotional health in general, in relation to the interaction of the barriers.

*

IN SUMMARY

The outside world comes in and is filtered in so many ways. It is filtered through our intestinal epithelial barrier, the blood-enteric barrier, the blood-brain barrier, our emotional history and life experience expressed in our cells and in tissue memory, epigenetics, our in-utero and birth experiences emotionally, chemically, and physically, and the epigenetics and molecular memories passed down to us through generations. Our bodies are complex and connected on every level—emotional, mental, physical, chemical, and environmental—and our lives are not only imprinted by, but have

---

*The endoderm is the innermost germ layer that forms the linings of the respiratory and gastrointestinal tracts and their associated organs during embryonic development.
†The mesoderm is the middle layer of the three germ layers that develop during gastrulation in the very early development of the embryo of most animals. The outer layer is the ectoderm, and the inner layer is the endoderm. Mesoderm tissues are derived from the mesoderm.

also created, the body-mind experience we now have. Instead of despairing, the fact that everything can be influenced by everything we do and think from now onward, and that all changes, whether tiny or huge, will impact everything in us, from each cell to our whole mind-body-spirit, gives us power and hope. We are always a work in progress—all of us.

Case Story—Stephen
Working at the Cellular Level

Stephen was a little boy of fourteen months who came to see me because he was vomiting often. He had a poor appetite, and he was not putting on enough weight. Doctors had found nothing clinically "wrong" with him. He was a very active little boy.

The first time I treated Stephen, even with a box of delightful toys and a willing and helpful mother playing with him, it was quite tricky to touch him, especially on his head. Over the first few sessions, he became more willing to accept the work and would come into my room smiling and looking forward to playing. I spent most of the time on his tummy, releasing patterns of tension and restriction there. Something by the basement membrane once again called to me to work very specifically there with my intention and palpation to facilitate a more relaxed membrane.

Stephen was making good progress. His vomiting reduced greatly, and his appetite increased. But when we had a gap of six weeks between treatments, as I was away teaching, he retrogressed. Fortunately, this regression was not to where he began, but his vomiting certainly increased and appetite decreased.

His gut seemed hypersensitive and reacted strongly unless his nervous systems were calmed down. When I had my hands on him, I consistently worked my way down through the layers of the small intestine to contact the enteric nervous system and the many different cell groups that communicated with it and supported it.

I began to suspect some neurological issues, beginning in the enteric nervous system and, of course, then impacting the autonomic nervous system and the central nervous system. His mouth appeared to be very sensitive, and I imagined it holds much tension. (He had teeth and did not understand the concept of not biting the therapist, so I was not able to manage working there! I did work into the mouth from the outside, however.) I wonder, therefore, if he has some sensory integration issues.

After a few more sessions, his enteric system seemed to settle, and he progressed to consistent good appetite and eating with no vomiting. I see Stephen every few months, just because mum recognizes what a great support this work is for a growing child.

This Story's Message

Stephen illustrates how tension in the layers of his small intestine and possibly issues in the intestinal epithelial barrier can impact appetite, eating, and digestion.

11

Post-Traumatic Gut Disorder Lives

Today was not meant to be a writing day, but I am sitting here with a perfect example of Post-Traumatic Gut Disorder fresh in my mind. I know Post-Traumatic Gut Disorder is not really an official label, but I am putting it forward as a new way of describing what I have and continue to experience. I really want to know if it is familiar to any of you too. In fact, I would like to remove the "disorder" part from the label. Post-Traumatic Gut (or PTG) is a better option in my mind. A disorder implies there is something inherently wrong with a person rather than the person responding in a normal way to very intense and overwhelming experiences that they are struggling to integrate and live with. The label PTG also seems to leave the door more open for potential resolution.

Memories of PTG

A few days of challenge and my sleep and gut both respond with restlessness and burning sensations. A feeling of extreme fullness after eating supper, slight nausea, and anxiety lead me to a night where I wake with hot burning in my gut. A fire is sweeping—or so it seems—the top layer of skin from the lumen, traveling from my esophagus, through my stomach, and into my intestine. My mouth is parched and dry. Why, I wonder, is my body so angry with the outside world? The cells in the different tissues in my long tube are raging like a forest fire taking everything in its wake; sleep, peace, calm, all are gone for now. I have to get out of bed, drink cold water, and walk into the bathroom. Relishing the cold floor on my bare feet, I wait for the flames to subside. A little while later, I return to bed and, focusing on my breathing, slip into sleep once more. I repeat this process twice more that night. These nights are disturbing. The only thing that has changed is how I perceive them. Less resistance and more love is my ongoing intention, which brings emotion like a small stream of cool water flowing through the hot spaces.

Other times, there are no obvious triggers. Life seems kind, and yet, there is clearly unrest deep inside that surfaces sometimes. Trying to work out what is happening and why it is happening now is a thankless task. I have more acceptance of these events than I used to. Instead of struggling with the why, I focus on listening and breathing and allowing them to pass. The following is a typical example.

Another recent night, I went to bed feeling relaxed and dozy. I had a really great day off—I walked in the sun, did a little shopping, and went to a yoga workshop, followed by home-cooked supper with my husband and daughter. I curled up in bed and began to feel sleepy.

Nothing was stressing me, or so I thought—although there was a little feeling of being disconnected from my surroundings. I concentrated on the weight of my body on the bed beneath me. I focused on the sheets touching my skin. My body felt too light, too absent from me somehow.

This feeling of not being able to really feel stable in the room was very familiar to me and has been part of my PTG and anxiety for many years. I concentrated again on feeling the touch of the mattress and sheets underneath me. I opened my eyes to pick out tiny cracks of light through the shutters and take some comfort from the visual reference point that gave me. I closed my eyes again. Still somewhere between sleeping and waking, I felt a little dizzy and floaty. I wondered whether or not to open my eyes again but I was scared the room might be turning around me. (This has often happened in the past. Losing all stable visual reference in the outside world has been part of my deepest experience of post-traumatic stress and my gut's rapid descent into fight or flight.)

I opened my eyes very slowly and was relieved that the room was not turning, but I felt a switch suddenly go on in my body. My heart jumped into a pounding rhythm and adrenaline surged through my body, taking me violently into a state of fear. Strangely, fear is so familiar to me that I am no longer afraid of it flooding my system. Nausea rose, dizziness filled my head, and my gut started to cramp. My breath felt difficult. I had to get out of bed and walk. I drank water. My gut decided to get rid of any food waste it was still holding. My heart was still thumping, and I still felt really sick and wobbly. I had no idea why any of this was happening. It was not related to the present but to the past. That was all I knew. I felt as if I had been catapulted into space, attached by a tentative thread to this planet. My sense of my body was slipping out of my grasp, like water running through the fingers of my hand. The earth beneath me turned to shifting sands under my feet, as it had done so many times in the past. My mind was washed over by waves of uncertainty and curiosity, as if I were suddenly hurled into another universe where different natural laws apply.

Eventually, tiredness appeared again, and I got back into bed. Placing one hand on my solar plexus and the other on my small intestine, I focused on breathing and listening to my gut. I wanted it to be heard, to know that I was listening to what was happening, and to reassure all the cells there that I was not, in fact, in danger but was safe at home. Gradually I managed to fall asleep. On waking, I still felt wobbly inside, and my heart was still fluttering a little. Even some hours later in the afternoon, that feeling remained. These experiences tell me that memories in my body are triggered by many different things that I am not always aware of, that the sensitive response of my gut to stimuli is below the conscious part of my brain, or brains.

Sleep is often not my friend. For so many years there have been nights that are a restless search for peace, often with an array of discomfort—heart palpitations, gut cramps, burning in the tube, nausea, frequent bowel movements, dizziness, and disconnection. Much of this is accompanied by flashbacks of the scuba diving accident and relentless visits from that group of homeless children—my childhood memories—each carrying a part of my early experience in their hearts.

GROWING INTO YOUR NEW SELF

Sleep has a rhythm, taking our brain through different cycles in order to process our lives, cleanse our brain and other organs, and repair our bodies. There is a ninety-minute cycle of slow-wave sleep, followed by a period of rapid eye movement (REM) sleep where we often dream. During the night, while it is empty, the gut brain, our enteric nervous system, produces a ninety-minute slow wave of muscle contractions, followed by short bursts of rapid muscle movement. It appears that the two brains are linked in sleep, and individuals with bowel problems, such as myself, are found to have abnormal REM sleep. I have a sleep tracker that I wear at night, and I notice I have at least twice the normal amount of REM sleep and often reduced deep sleep. REM sleep is involved with processing experience and with creativity. The relationship between the two brains has much to teach us and leaves us with more questions than answers. The delicate balance of all the chemicals, neurotransmitters, and microbiota in this relationship can be so easily thrown out by our lives and also by medications that can create catastrophic cascades of dysfunction.

Memory is stored in the enteric nervous system, in the fascial layers of the gut, in the microbiota, and in the fluids. I have a picture of molecular footprints left in the sand of my body, as deep memories and intense emotion walk side by side along the edge of the ocean where water meets land. Once again, I find the key to understanding resides between two worlds, the water and the land, the past and the present, the place where the lumen meets my inner world.

This idea reminds me of that pivotal meeting several years after the onset of my PTSD. I mentioned this briefly before. I had a spectacular piece of advice from the third cardiologist I saw after my scuba diving accident. He was a man of great compassion, and at that time in my recovery, he turned everything around for me with these words: "Do not try to be the person you were before that event. Discover who you are now." These words have stayed with me ever since and I am forever grateful to him for his humanity and wisdom. He supported me as I came off the anti-arrhythmia drugs that were turning me into a zombie, and I told him I intended to take up yoga instead. His door was always open. He created a space in which I could begin to heal. He introduced me to the idea of Post-Traumatic Growth, although I would not have recognized this as a concept at the time. It was an idea that with the suffering, anxiety, and depression that comes in the aftermath of trauma, there is the possibility of growth.

Gradually, I am learning to stop fighting the world coming into me on every level. Instead of seeing the ideal form of myself that I would like to create and feeling disappointed and ashamed of the reality that is me now, I am learning more compassion for myself. I embrace the many influences on my whole mind-body-spirit from previous generations, my childhood experiences, and my near drowning as an enriching part of the person I am now. I embrace too the complex emotional experience I often live with—the vagaries of my sleep and digestion—instead of fighting every discomfort. In particular, I am learning to listen to my gut without seeing it or feeling it as an adversary.

I have become aware that I was receiving the outside world into my gut with distrust, suspicion, and guardedness by responding through the filter of all that had been. I have also become aware that this was deeply hidden for a long time below my rational brain and my heart. Gradually, I am more able to listen to the stories in my second brain with acceptance and kindness. This has helped my gut feel more resilient and comfortable. I am learning to appreciate my body, my health, and the fact that I am still alive and that each day is a gift. I am learning to appreciate that even when I do not feel so bouncy, and even when my gut feels sore, it is completely possible to find joy and happiness both inside me and around me.

As Albert Camus once said, "In the depths of winter, I finally learned that within me there lay an invincible summer."

The whole person that I am, that you are, is a complicated mix of past and present, and that mix is perfect, and so are we. Perfect in our imperfection. Look around at everything in nature—every tree, every flower in bloom—and see all the imperfections of shape and asymmetries in color, size, and finish. Pause for a moment to wonder what the world would be like if these were all the same, all "perfect." How uninteresting and bland nature would be to our eyes! Why apply a different set of rules to humankind? How can we tune into the riches of our individual complexity?

FIELD THEORY

This takes me back to field theory, which is discussed in the areas of psychology and sociology. It describes how we interact as individuals with our social context and how our field will align itself with the social or organizational context we find ourselves in. It is discussed as well in the area of physics, especially quantum physics. My colleague Tad Wanveer has posed the question of whether the glial matrix in the brain in the head may be part of the greater physical field in which we live on this planet and in this universe.

The glial matrix in our brain is a responsive and activating network, and perhaps this interacts with the greater field outside us. Likewise, the glial cells in our enteric nervous system are perhaps interacting with the field outside too. I am seeing the interwoven body we inhabit—and particularly our glial selves—expanding, contracting, weaving, and distorting as the whole constantly adapts and responds in a fluid and plastic way to the life in and around us. In my mind's eye, it is a continuously shifting flow. Adaptation contains all the complexities of the many different extraordinary cells and bacteria within the human body, both influencing and being influenced by them. I picture it as a field at one with the universal field, and I realize this is my own idea and fantasy, but that is how it feels to my body-mind complex.

If the ideas above are true of the glial matrix in the brain in the head, why would it not be true of the glial matrix in our enteric nervous system in our gut? If this is the case, are we both influencing and influenced by the greater field around us in a fluid and neurological way?

How does all this relate to our neuroplasticity and glial plasticity? And what impact does this neuroplasticity and glial plasticity have on our personal field? There are an extraordinary number of influences on our personal field through environmental, emotional, chemical, and intergenerational experiences. We can reflect on how complex the influences on each individual's field must be and how equally complex the individual's influence out into the greater field must also be. Human beings are mostly in an impossible struggle to be neutral.

SEEKING NEUTRALITY AS A THERAPIST

Pondering ideas of neuroplasticity, glial plasticity, and field theory brings me to our work as Upledger CranioSacral therapists. We intend and strive to be grounded, blended, and neutral. But how can we become neutral? By doing our own inner work to become as aware as possible of all the complex influences on us and therefore on our field, we can be a little clearer and therefore more helpful to our clients. This is the big challenge.

Recognizing the complexity of each individual is also the reason that protocols and agendas in treatment often fail. By doing our own work, being fully present and aware in our own body-field, and blending with another's field and listening to him or her with as neutral a pair of hands as possible, we can help facilitate his or her healing.

When we blend with the person on the table, does our field align with theirs? This seems very likely to me.

TOLERATING UNCERTAINTY

As we come nearer to the end of our journey together within these pages, I feel that something is not right. Surely this book about the gut, my gut in particular, should end with my triumphant declaration of having the perfect bowel. That is how it was meant to be, wasn't it?

Instead, I am sitting here with a tender gut, low energy, and a slightly low mood after a night of, shall we say, enthusiastic peristalsis. Even more ironic is the fact that it is probably this part of the book that triggered the gut episode. Anxious about what to say next, anxious about how helpful it will be to anyone, anxious about how to draw it all together, and now anxious because my gut is clearly not "fixed"!

I am moving away from the idea or goal of fixing myself, of finding clear labels or diagnoses, as I become aware of the complexity that is me and, of course, you. It feels as if tolerating uncertainty is important and realistic. Interestingly, I have found a recent piece of research titled "Tolerating Uncertainty—The Next Medical Revolution?"[47] The research team begins by quoting John Keats, 1817: "At once it struck me what quality went to form a Man of Achievement . . . when a man is capable of being in uncertainties, mysteries, doubts, without any irritable reaching after fact and reason."

Keats was a poet and also a physician. In medicine and health care today, there is a drive toward making a diagnosis, being rational and fact driven, and definitely not appearing uncertain or unknowing of an answer. This drive can be restricting, misleading, and misguiding. This team of researchers is encouraging a new culture in health, where uncertainty and curiosity are tolerated and embraced, and all is not black and white. They feel the next medical revolution depends on this shift. They feel that medical training would benefit from a curriculum that recognizes diagnosis as dynamic, evolving, and inclusive of the patient's perspective. Perhaps hypotheses would be a better word in the future than diagnosis, thereby changing the expectations of both patients and physicians. They end by saying that certainty is an illusion. I am including this study as it resonates with the approach that we as Upledger CranioSacral therapists have to the people that come to us. Personally, letting go of certainty has helped me in my own health and in my clinical practice. It is all a journey, after all.

I experience another big difference between then and now, between the two worlds of past trauma and current reality. This is compassion for myself, an expanded awareness of what my past experience has created and a better capacity to listen to the many, often-confused messages my body and, in particular, my gut are sending me. This has been made possible by the physicians, therapists, family, and friends who have held space for me, without trying to provide answers, to go on my journey toward better health.

Sharing my story has been a big part of my evolution. I am sharing my humanity with you and offering all of myself, without excuse or apology, steady in my vulnerability, and reaching out with compassion to you, dear reader.

Case Story—Jane
The Potential for Transformation

In Jane's own words: "I first started seeing Nikki after her colleague suggested she could help me with my digestion issues. I have a connective tissue disorder, Ehlers Danlos Syndrome, which affects collagen production, and therefore the whole body. I suffer from dysmotility in my digestive system, which leaves me with symptoms of nausea, bloating, pain, cramping, and constipation. When Nikki started working on me, after a few minutes, I started to feel my stomach relax and I got a feeling I can only describe as 'sloshing'! My usual gurgling, painful, and angry stomach started to transform into one with satisfactory rumbling and soft, loose muscles! After my sessions, I experienced full-body relaxation and drowsiness. I slept brilliantly that night, which made a change from my insomnia-filled nights! Part of my dysmotility is my stomach empties very slowly. I am nasogastric-tube dependent for all my nutrition, and to check if it is in the correct place, I must aspirate the tube. Usually, I get a test of food, but after a session of CranioSacral Therapy, I got clear bile. The effects usually last around twenty-four hours."

Jane is a teenager with severe Ehlers Danlos Syndrome, which results in her being almost unable to walk or hold her head up. She experiences very painful dislocation of joints throughout her body and enormous digestive issues. Jane cannot swallow anything except water and is fed through a nasogastric tube. Even this method of feeding takes hours, as she is unable to tolerate more than a very slow feed without experiencing extreme nausea and bloating. Her abdomen can bloat up to ten inches during just one feed, and she is always severely constipated, as her gut motility is very poor. Her dream is to be able to eat and digest her food more normally and not have to use the nasogastric tube.

Jane's body is a complex mixture of laxity and extreme tension. Not surprisingly, her anxiety levels are very high, as she has to deal with so much dysfunction while maintaining her education and her normal teenage friendships.

Back when I evaluated her system as I always do, I was directed to her gut. Putting my hands on it, I felt a stillness and tension there. I simply listened with soft, neutral hands and waited for the tissue to engage with me and begin to unwind. After a while, this happened, and there was relaxation, warmth, and much gurgling that delighted both Jane and myself. Jane commented on how relaxed her gut felt compared with how it normally felt. After that session, she and her mother reported she had a big feed with very little nausea and no bloating at all. Wow!

After three sessions, Jane and her mother reported that they noticed after a treatment that her stomach was completely empty. Normally, it takes many hours for food to go through her stomach. They were able to notice the change because they use a syringe to draw up fluid from her stomach (through the end of the tube that is placed there) before feeding her to see how acidic her stomach is, and check that the tube is in the right place. Normally, there would be some of the food in the syringe too, as the stomach would not have emptied properly. However, after three sessions, her stomach was emptying properly. Now, after each session, when they do the syringe check, there is no food left in it.

This effect is currently temporary, but it shows what is possible, and I am confident it will continue to improve. I taught Jane some hands-on work she can do, which was challenging for her, as her digestive system had not been her friend for a long time, but she was open-minded and willing to go on that journey.

In time, Jane made huge progress and showed great courage in her journey. She is now walking without crutches or the support of a walking stick, has no feeding tube and is eating practically normally, and is off many of her pain killers. She attended art college. Incredible! What an honor to witness!

This Story's Message

Jane came to me with a diagnosis of Ehlers Danlos Syndrome (EDS), unable to eat or move out of bed. Her EDS and accompanying psychological issues are complex, and she is a good illustration of how, as therapists, we need to respond to the unique individual in front of us with a beginner's mind. An illustration of always holding the space for potential transformation.

12

So, What Now?

How to Go from Dis-ease to Ease in the Gut

All disease begins in the gut.
HIPPOCRATES

This book has been all about expanding your awareness of what can influence the health of your gut and how the gut remembers your life experiences. It is about casting the net much wider than looking at the food on our plate. Nutrition is an important part of the journey—clean eating is important—but, to a large extent, the emotional history in our gut will define how we receive what comes into the long tube in terms of food, chemicals, and additives. We are all so individual and respond to all of these in a unique way. There is no formula for diet; there is only your own gut with its own history. Find a nutritionist who recognizes this and will work with you on your own journey. Finally, it is about offering you a way forward by empowering you with information, enabling a better connection with the stories in your gut, and suggesting strategies that may help you work with all of this.

Looking back, I realize that there are lots of ideas and strategies scattered among the previous chapters. Even so, you may still be wondering how to make a plan from all of that information. So here are my suggestions for creating a peaceful gut, or at least for setting off on that journey.

My first recommendation is that you give yourself some time to consider and reflect on any traumatic events or experiences, challenges, or periods of chronic stress in your life, your parents' lives, your grandparents' lives, or your children's lives. As we have seen from the research on epigenetics, cell memory and multigenerational influences have potent influence on your gut health.

Your emotional experience is the single biggest influence on your mental and physical health, and your second brain responds instantly. Remember, the outside world comes into your body via the long tube. Notice how you tend to respond to the outside world. Is your response always calm and relaxed and adaptive? Or does it tend to be guarded and tense or you react with panic and fear?

Trauma and difficult emotional experiences leave a memory and a trail of influence in the gut, its second brain, and its microbiome—which in turn influences your first brain with the central nervous system and your overall health. This is the root of ill health in the gut and therefore the whole body.

Next, consider your stress levels, both now and in the past. Is there a gap between what is expected of you and what you feel able to achieve? This is the space filled with stress, and many people spend much of their lives in a state of stress. Stress, as we have seen, impacts the gut immediately and negatively and eats away at your resilience and ability to bounce back from challenges in your life. Sometimes it is difficult to change everything in your life that produces stress, but you can control how you respond to it and how you build your resources accordingly.

For the whole continuum of everyday stress into extreme personal and family trauma, the following are ways to help yourself.

Do Your Inner Work!

This is top of the list for a reason. It is the single biggest factor in your mental and physical health, and that health begins in the gut. Emotional work will help you become aware of, express, and integrate deeply held experiences and patterns in a way that reduces their power and influence over your health by releasing tension and imbalance in your body-mind system.

How do you do this? One very potent way is through Upledger CranioSacral Therapy with its associated SomatoEmotional Release techniques that I have described in the earlier chapters. These techniques are such an incredible way to access emotion and trauma buried deep in the tissues of your body and to allow it to release naturally and gently. Much of these experiences are found in the gut, and that is why I have written this book, to help us listen to the stories written there.

Other forms of therapy, such as acupuncture, counseling, and other types of bodywork—visceral manipulation, lymphatic drainage, myofascial work, and massage—can also be very helpful in moving you forward. Without this work, optimal health in the gut and elsewhere will always be an impossible dream. Often, a mixture of different kinds of input at different times is effective. Trust what feels right for you now, and give it a chance to help by having a few sessions.

Breathe

Learn to breathe! Sounds crazy? Surely, I am breathing all the time. Well, yes and no! Many of us breathe shallowly and without expanding our lungs or our whole thoracic area. Unless you breathe well and mindfully, your vagus nerve will not be able to function well and nor will your gut. (Remember vagal tone's big connection with the gut, resilience, managing stress, and reducing tension in your neck and shoulders?) Find a meditation or mindfulness class and learn to breathe well.

Conscious breathing also connects the mind with the body, thus building your ability to listen to the messages from the body. In this case, the gut is sending you, through interoception, your felt sense of your inner world. Breath can be a huge part of your journey of seeking connection with yourself and of integrating your experiences.

One very simple way of breathing is to spend a few minutes every day, or a few minutes several times a day, doing conscious breathing. All you do is silently say to yourself "I am breathing in" on your breath in and then "I am breathing out" on your breath out. In this way, your mind will find it gradually easier to focus on your breathing. Other thoughts and ideas will quite naturally come into your awareness, and that is okay; just keep coming back to your conscious breathing.

Be even more specific once you are more connected to your breath by resting your hands on your gut and breathing into your hands gently and mindfully. Listen very carefully with your hands to any tensions, emotions, or other sensations or lack of sensations you notice by doing this.

If you are sitting or lying down with your hands on your gut while breathing, you could also gently massage the abdomen with your hands clockwise and then counterclockwise, sending it whatever you feel it might need—calm, peace, love, reassurance, or compassion.

Try Intentioned Touch

Earlier in this book (p. 32) I suggested you might like to lie or sit with your hands on your gut and send your intention with your hands through the many layers of the small intestine and bowel. By using a soft touch with listening hands and focusing on one layer at a time, it could offer you an experience full of insight into your gut health and therefore your whole health.

Here are the layers again to remind you:

- Skin
- Superficial fascia under the skin
- Mesentery
- Longitudinal Muscle
- Auerbach's or Myenteric Nerve Plexus
- Circular Muscle
- Submucosal layer
- Mucosa
  - Lamina propria
  - Basement membrane
  - Villi
  - Epithelium
- Lumen

Use a Tummy Tracker Journal

These notebooks are carefully designed to track the different factors that might impact your gut function and health. They are small enough to carry in your bag and detailed enough to make sure you do not forget anything. Be consistent about your tummy tracking and you may begin to see a pattern or notice triggers that have never been in your awareness before.

Notice What Triggers a Reaction in Your Gut

The trigger might be a food, a thought, a relationship, a work stress, a memory, or many other things. Give yourself time to reflect on this and consider ways of eliminating, reducing, or responding differently to that stressor or trigger.

Build Resilience to Stress

You can build resilience to stress in numerous ways, such as those noted below.

Breathing—Breathing is essential for gut health, vagal tone, and building resilience to stress.

Singing—Singing is wonderful for breathing, relaxing, expressing, literally finding our voice, and moving the respiratory diaphragm. Singing in a choir is a fantastic way to connect with other people, which adds to its stress-busting capability.

Yoga—Yoga is one of the strategies recommended by a leading expert in the field of trauma and post-traumatic stress, Bessel van der Kolk, in his integrated approach to trauma.[48] It is a way of allowing us to make a friend of our body once more—a total body-mind system for transforming ourselves into calm, happy folk. Find a kind of yoga that suits you from the many types:

- Ashtanga yoga—for the fit and dynamic folk who crave movement to relax
- Vinyasa Flow—for a more dance-like sequencing of moves, with emphasis on breath, strength, and flexibility
- Hatha yoga—for a gentler, less dynamic experience that is also great for beginners

- Yin yoga—where postures are held for a long time to allow us to fully breathe into our tight spaces and give the fascia and connective tissue time to let go
- Restorative yoga—for total bliss, relaxation, or rehabilitation after illness, again giving the body time to let go in supported asanas (postures)

Meditation and Mindfulness—Both of these help us breathe and be present in the now, rather than anxious about the past or the future.

Tai Chi—Tai Chi is graceful, builds balance and strength, and calms. It is a wonderful way to relax the spine and the central nervous system.

Dancing or any other kind of movement—The body loves to move. The gut bacteria need us to be active in order to be healthy. If they are not healthy, neither are we.

Walking—Just going for a walk outside in the fresh air for half an hour each day is a huge support for the health of the gut. Our gut bacteria love being taken for a walk.

Laughter—Laughter is emotional release; it helps you breathe, loosens the diaphragm, and brings relaxation to the gut. You can never have too much.

Eat well—There are many highly qualified and skilled nutritionists out there who can advise on foods that are healthy for you as an individual and on those that are not. I would just say, eat a wide range of high-quality, unprocessed foods (foods without a list of ingredients on the label!), and drink plenty of water each day.

Anything that makes you smile, laugh, feel relaxed, and happy—Do more of this regularly.

✳

So it is time to part company, you and I. I hope you have enjoyed the journey and that you will explore your gut issues with curiosity and compassion now.

Healing ourselves or making ourselves whole by integrating our experiences through self-awareness is the process that will take us to the ultimate goal of therapy, which is self-realization.

APPENDIX

Tummy Tracker

On the next page is a prompt to help you start the important work of tracking all the elements that are affecting your gut health on your journey toward better physical and emotional health.

A journal of tummy tracker pages that I designed is available from the Upledger Institute's website and the International Alliance of Healthcare Educators' website.

If your gut could make a face
RIGHT NOW,
what would it look like?
Trace the circle below and draw that face inside it to see what your
gut is trying to tell you. Then consider the prompts below.

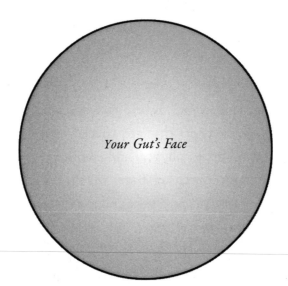

Your Gut's Face

What foods did you eat?

How are you feeling:
Mentally?

Physically?

Emotionally?

References

1. John E. Upledger, *Your Inner Physician and You* (Berkeley: North Atlantic Books, 1992).

2. Kate Mackinnon, *From My Hands and Heart: Achieving Health and Balance with CranioSacral Therapy* (Carlsbad, Calif., Hay House, 2013).

3. J. Calvin Coffey and D. Peter O'Leary, "The Mesentery, Structure, Function and Role in Disease," *The Lancet Gastroenterology and Hepatology* 1 (2016): 238–42.

4. V. J. Felliti, R. F. Anda, D. Nordenberg, D. Williamson, A. M. Spitz, V. Edwards, M. P. Koss, and J. S. Marks, "Relationship of Childhood Abuse and Household Dysfunction to Many of the Leading Causes of Death in Adults: The Adverse Childhood Experiences (ACE) Study," *American Journal of Preventative Medicine* 14, no. 4 (1998): 245–58.

5. Norman Doidge, *The Brain That Changes Itself* (New York: Viking Press, 2007).

6. M. C. Diamon, A. B. Scheibel, G. M. Murphy Jr., and T. Harvey, "On the Brain of a Scientist: Albert Einstein," *Experimental Neurology* 88, no. 1 (April 1985): 198–204.

7. Tad Wanveer, *Brain Stars: Glia Illuminating CranioSacral Therapy* (Palm Beach Gardens, Fla.: Upledger Institute, 2005).

8. Michael Morgan, *The Body Energy Longevity Prescription: How CranioSacral Therapy Helps Prevent Alzheimer's and Dementia While Improving the Quality of Your Life* (Fairfield, Iowa: The Body Energy Company, 2014).

9. Jennifer Labus, Emily B. Hollister, Jonathan Jacobs, Kyleigh Kirbach, Numan Oezguen, Arpana Gupta, Jonathan Acosta, et al., "Differences in Gut Microbial Composition Correlate with Regional Brain Volumes in Irritable Bowel Syndrome," *Microbiome* 5, no. 49 (2017).

10. Steven Porges, *Polyvagal Theory* (New York: W. Norton and Company, 2011).

11. Steven Porges and Senta A. Furman, "The Early Development of the Autonomic Nervous System Provides a Neural Platform for Social Behavior: A Polyvagal Perspective," *Infant and Child Development* 20, no. 1 (2011): 106–18.

12. Rachel Yehuda, Nikolaos P. Daskalakis, Linda M. Bierer, Heather N. Bader, Torsten Klengel, Florian Holsboer, and Elisabeth Binder, "Holocaust Induced Intergenerational Effects on $FKBP_5$ Methylation," *Biological Psychiatry* 80, no. 5 (September 2016): 376–80.

13. Brian G. Dias and Kerry J. Ressler, "Parental Olfactory Experience Influences Behaviour and Neural Structure in Subsequent Generations," *Nature Neuroscience* 17 (2013): 89–96.

14. Jamie A. Hackett, Roopsha Sengupta, Jan J. Zylicz, Kazuhiro Murakami, Caroline Lee, Thomas A. Down, and M. Azim Surani, "Germline DNA Demethylation Dynamics and Imprint Erasure through 5-Hydroxymethlcytosine," *Science* 339, no. 6118 (2013): 448–52.

15. Katharina Gapp, Ali Jawaid, Peter Sarkies, Johannes Bohacek, Pawel Pelczar, Julien Prados, Laurent Farinelli, Eric Miska, and Isabelle M. Mansuy, "Implication of Sperm RNAs in Transgenerational Inheritance of the Effects of Early Trauma in Mice," *Nature Neuroscience* 17, no. 17 (2014): 667–69.

16. Adam Klosin, Eduard Casas, Cristina Hidalgo-Carcedo, Tanya Vavouri, and Ben Lehner, "Transgenerational Transmission of Environmental Information in C. Elegans," *Science* 356, no. 6335 (2017): 320–23.

17. Torsten Santavirta, Nina Santavirta, and Stephen Gilman, "Association of the World War II Finnish Evacuation of Children with Psychiatric Hospitalization in the Next Generation," *Jama Psychiatry* 3511 (2017): 21–27.

18. Steven Porges and Senta A. Furman, "The Early Development of the Autonomic Nervous System Provides a Neural Platform for Social Behavior: A Polyvagal Perspective," *Infant and Child Development* 20, no. 1 (2011): 106–18.

19. Robert K. Naviaux, "Metabolic Features of the Cell Danger Response," *Mitochondrian* 16 (2014): 7–17.

20. Ulrike Ehlert, "Enduring Psychobiological Effects of Childhood Adversity," *Psychoneuroendocrinology* 38, no. 9 (2013): 1850–57.

21. Joseph L. Edmonds, Daniel J. Kirse, Donald Kearns, Reena Deutsch, Liesbeth Spruijt, and Robert K. Naviaux, "The Otolaryngological Manifestations of Mitochondrial Disease and the Risk of Neurodegeneration with Infection," *Archives of Otorhinolaryngology—Head & Neck Surgery* 128, no. 4 (2002): 355–62.

22. Thomas P. Chapman, Gina Hadley, Carl Fratter, Sue N. Cullen, Bridget E. Bax, Murray D. Bain, Robert A. Sapsford, Joanna Poulton, and Simon P. Travis, "Unexplained Gastrointestinal Symptoms: Think Mitochondrial Disease," *Digestive and Liver Disease* 46, no. 1 (2014): 1–8.

23. Robert K. Naviaux, "Mitochondrial Control of Epigenetics," *Cancer Biology & Therapy* (2008): 1191–93.

24. Katharina Austen, Pia Ringer, Alexander Mehlich, Anna Chrostek-Grashoff, Carleen Kluger, Christoph Klinger, Benedikt Sabass, Roy Zent, Matthias Rief, and Carsten Grashoff, "Extracellular Rigidity Sensing by Talin Isoform-Specific Mechanical Linkages," *Nature Cell Biology* 17 (2015): 1597–606.

25. Arash Tajik, Yuejin Zhang, Fuxiang Wei, Jian Sun, Qiong Jia, Wenwen Zou, Rishi Singh, Nimish Khanna, Andrew S. Belmont, and Ning Wang, "Transcription Upregulation via Force-Induced Direct Stretching of Chromatin," *Nature Materials* 15 (2016): 1287–96.

26. Franziska Denk, Meghan Crow, Athanasios Didangelos, Douglas M. Lopes, and Stephen B. McMahon, "Persistent Alterations in Microglial Enhancers in a Model of Chronic Pain," *CellPress* 15, no. 8 (2016): 1771–81.

27. J. B. Furness, N. Clerc, and W. A. A. Kunze, "Memory in the Enteric Nervous System," *BMJ GUT* 47, no. 4 (2000).

28. Roland Mathis and Martin Ackermann, "Response of Single Bacterial Cells to Stress Gives Rise to Complex History Dependence at the Population Level," *PNAS* 113, no. 15 (2016): 4224–29.

29. EAWAG: Swiss Federal Institute of Aquatic Science and Technology, "Collective Memory Discovered in Bacteria," Science Daily website (March 7, 2016).

30. Ravinarayan Raghupathi, Michael D. Duffield, Leah Zelkas, Adrian Meedeniya, Simon J. H. Brookes, Tiong Cheng Sia, David A. Wattchow, Nick J. Spencer, and Damien J. Keating, "Identification of Unique Release Kinetics of Serotonin from Guinea-Pig and Human Enterochromaffin Cells," *The Journal of Physiology* 591, no. 23 (Dec. 1, 2013): 5959–75.

31. Christopher S. Reigstad, Charles E. Salmonson, John F. Rainey III, Joseph H. Szurszewski, David R. Linden, Justin L. Sonnenburg, Gianrico Farrugia, and Purna C. Kashyap, "Gut Microbes Promote Colonic Serotonin Production through an Effect of Short-Chain Fatty Acids on Enterochromaffin Cells," *The FASEB Journal* 29, no. 4 (Apr. 2015): 1395–1403.

32. Magdy El-Salhy, Doris Gundersen, Odd Helge Gilja, Jan Gunnar Hatlebakk, and Trygve Hausken, "Is Irritable Bowel Syndrome an Organic Disorder?" *World Journal of Gastroenterology* 20, no. 2 (2014): 384–400.

33. Marcus Manocha and Waliul I. Khan, "Serotonin and GI Disorders: An Update on Clinical and Experimental Studies," *Clinical and Translational Gastroenterology* 3, no. 13 (2012).

34. Diego V. Bohórquez, Leigh A. Samsa, Andrew Roholt, Satish Medicetty, Rashmi Chandra, and Rodger A. Liddle, "An Enteroendocrine Cell–Enteric Glia Connection Revealed by 3D Electron Microscopy," *PLOS One* 9, no. 2 (2014).

35. Werend Boesmars, Michiel A. Martens, Nathalie Weltens, Marlene M. Hao, Jan Tack, Carla Cirillo, and Pieter Vanden Berghe, "Imaging Neuron-Glia Interaction in Enteric Nervous System," *Front Cell Neuroscience* 21 (2013): 183.

36. Keith A. Sharkey, "Emerging Roles for Enteric Glia in Gastrointestinal Disorders," *Journal of Clinical Investigation* 121, no. 9 (2011): 3412–24.

37. Fernando Ochoa-Cortes, Fabio Turco, Andromeda Linan-Rico, Suren Soghomonyan, Emmett Whitaker, Sven Wehner, Rosario Cuomo, and Fievos L. Christofi, "Enteric Glial Cells: A New Frontier in Neurogastroenterology and Clinical Target for Inflammatory Bowel Disease," *PUBMED* 22, no. 2 (2016): 433–49.

38. Luisa Seguella and Brian D. Gulbransen, "Enteric Glial Biology, Intercellular Signalling and Roles in Gastrointestinal Disease," *Nature Reviews Gastroenterology Hepatology* 18, no. 8 (March 17, 2021): 571–87.

39. Catia Laranjeira, Katarina Sandgren, Nicoletta Kessaris, William Richardson, Alexandre Potocnik, Pieter Vanden Berghe, Vassilis Pachnis, "Glial Cells in the Mouse Enteric Nervous System Can Undergo Neurogenesis in Response to Injury," *Journal of Clinical Investigation* 121, no. 9 (2011): 3412–24.

40. Luisa Seguella and Brian D. Gulbransen, "Enteric Glial Biology, Intercellular Signalling and Roles in Gastrointestinal Disease," *Nature Reviews Gastroenterology Hepatology* 18, no. 8 (March 17, 2021): 571–87.

41. Jacob M. Allen, Amy R. Mackos, Robert M. Jaggers, Patricia C. Brewster, Mikaela Webb, Chia-Hao Lin, Chris Ladaika, Ronald Davies, Peter White, Brett R. Loman, and Michael T. Bailey, "Psychological Stress Disrupts Intestinal Epithelial Cell Function and Mucosal Integrity through Microbe and Host-Directed Processes," *Gut Microbes* 14, no. 1 (2022).

42. Panagiotis S. Kabouridis and Vassilis Pachnis, "Emerging Roles of Gut Microbiota and the Immune System in the Development of the Enteric Nervous System," *Journal of Clinical Investigation* 125, no. 3 (March 2, 2015): 956–64.

43. Ilaria Spadoni, Elena Zagato, Alice Bertocchi, Roberta Paolinelli, Edina Hot, Antonio Di Sabatino, Flavio Caprioli, Luca Bottiglieri, Amanda Oldani, Giuseppe Viale, Giuseppe Penna, Elisabetta Dejana, and Maria Rescigno, "A Gut Vascular Barrier Controls the Systemic Dissemination of Bacteria," *Science* 350, no. 6262 (2015): 830–34.

44. Gen Zheng, Gordon Victor Fon, Walter Meixner, Amy Creekmore, Ye Zong, Michael K. Dame, Justin Colacino, Priya H. Dedhia, Shuangsong Hong, and John W. Wiley, "Chronic Stress and Intestinal Barrier Dysfunction," *Nature* 4502 (2017).

45. Sid Becker and Andrey Kuznetsov, eds., *Transport in Biological Media* (Amsterdam: Elsevier 2013).

46. Richard Daneman and Maria Rescigno, "The Gut Barrier and the Blood Brain Barrier: Are They So Different?" *Cell Immunity Review* 31, no. 5 (2009): 722–35.

47. Arabella L. Simpkin and Richard M. Schwartzstein, "Tolerating Uncertainty—The Next Medical Revolution?" *The New England Journal of Medicine* 375 (2016): 1713–15.

48. Bessel van der Kolk, *The Body Keeps the Score: Brain, Mind, and Body in the Healing of Trauma* (New York: Viking Penguin, 2014).

Index

About the Author

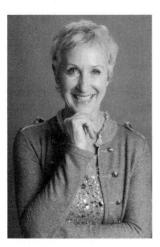

Nikki Kenward is an Upledger CranioSacral therapist with nearly twenty-five years of experience in private practice for adults, children, and babies. She teaches and examines internationally for the Upledger Institute and the International Alliance of Healthcare Educators (IAHE).

Nikki worked as a contemporary dancer, teacher, choreographer, and dance therapist for twenty-five years. Her dance work in the community took her into prisons with young male offenders, centers for people with chronic mental health issues, and eventually to create a dance theater company whose talented performers were all adults with learning difficulties. This company devised contemporary, movement-based, multisensory performances that toured to full houses.

Also a poet, Nikki has created a collection of poems that focus on emotional process and bodywork. As she wanted to include her creative work in her life again, Nikki recently completed an M.A. in Directing Circus. She is intending to extend her dance theater experience into contemporary circus to create work for diverse performers.

PRODUCTS OF RELATED INTEREST

Tummy Tracker Journal

This handy journal is full of blank gut faces to fill in on a daily or weekly basis. They have space opposite to note how you are emotionally, mentally, and physically, as well as anything else that seems at all relevant. Maintaining the journal assists you in seeing your patterns to help make positive adjustments in your life.

Wall Chart of the Second Brain: Understand Your Gut and Achieve Better Health

This chart is a valuable tool designed to support therapists in introducing their clients to the complexity and relevance of the gut to their health. Hung on the therapist's wall, it's a great starting point for a conversation and helps those clients with chronic digestive issues gain insight into this incredible system. It is often also used by colonic hydrotherapists to help show the gut's complexity and beauty.

Find these and more at your source for quality educational materials:
Upledger.com

FIND A PRACTITIONER

Upledger Institute International has trained healthcare practitioners in more than 110 countries. These include physical therapists, occupational therapists, massage therapists, chiropractors, osteopaths, medical doctors, naturopathic physicians, acupuncturists, and other body workers.

Many Upledger practitioners are members of the International Association of Healthcare Practitioners (IAHP).

Find a healthcare practitioner near you:
IAHP.com